We All Become Stories

The stories in this book are based on the experiences of the
author. Names and images of actual persons living or dead have been
altered out of consideration for privacy.

Illustrations by Jennifer Kenneally

Cover Design—Joanna Joseph/Typeset in Calibri and Garamond

Library and Archives Canada Cataloguing in Publication

Carson, Ann Elizabeth, 1929-, author
    We all become stories / Ann Elizabeth Carson ; illustrations by
Jennifer Kenneally. -- First edition.

Issued in print and electronic formats.
ISBN 978-0-9881478-2-9 (pbk.).--ISBN 978-0-9881478-4-3 (epub).--
ISBN 978-0-9881478-5-0 (kindle)

    1. Older people--Conduct of life--Anecdotes. 2. Aging--Anecdotes.
I. Kenneally, Jennifer, illustrator II. Title.

HQ1061.C37 2013   305.26   C2013-903884-1   C2013-903885-X

We All Become Stories

Ann Elizabeth Carson

Illustrations by Jennifer Kenneally

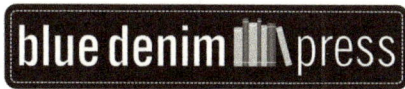

blue denim press

Ann Elizabeth Carson

December 2020

We All Become Stories is a memory bank opened to reveal the wisdom mined from experiences deeply felt and explored. These courageous discussions of what keeps the narrators alert, creative, loved and loving demonstrate how we learn along the way to feed our inner world. What sustains us in old age is what is absorbed earlier in life, not rote learning, but the storing of sensory memory and the gift of retrieving it. Read *We All Become Stories* and start to prepare now for a more fulfilling lifetime.

— Olive Senior, author of *Dancing Lessons* (Cormorant Books, 2011)

Yes, we all become stories—but it takes a poet to retell them in beautifully crafted prose and poetry. Carson's stories give voices to the silence that surrounds the reality of aging, especially in our time, and her poetry makes palpable the fleeting essence that all of us are.

— Max Layton, poet, singer-songwriter, author of *When The Rapture Comes* (Guernica Editions, 2012)

Ann Elizabeth Carson enters the room and her energy is alluring; she shows no sign of slowing down in her 80s. In *We All Become Stories*, Ann captures the sounds and the souls of 12 ordinary people who make extraordinary changes in their lives to find a place in a society that seldom honours old age. In prose as clear as polished crystal and a voice both brave and often humorous, Carson invites us to see ourselves in the past, present, and future through the words and hearts of elders whose moving stories will inspire you and leave you wiser for having read them.

— Gianni Patriarca, poet and storyteller, author of *Too Much Love* (Quattro Press, 2013)

Ann Elizabeth Carson makes us a great gift with her stories of our elders. She speaks with affection, compassion, insight, and spiritual depth of people who have endured much and learned much and have much to offer. Exploring with her and them the ways that memory changes and deepens, we discover that aging is an adventure that can be liberating and empowering for all of us who are treading paths into an uncertain future.

— Linda Stitt, poet, author of *Acting My Age* (2013)

Carson is serving as storycatcher here — deeply listening so that elders can formulate their own aging life story and deeply reflecting and telling her own aging life stories.

– Ellen B. Ryan, Ph.D., Professor Emeritus, McMaster University
www.writingdownouryears.ca

Also by Ann Elizabeth Carson:

Shadows Light, poetry and sculptures
My Grandmother's Hair, how family stories shape our memories and our lives
The Risks of Remembrance, new poems

For Margaret Ringer Howell

The world lives in order to develop lines in its face.

— T.E. Hulme

Table of Contents

Foreword: Listening

The world lives in order to develop lines in its face.
— T.E. Hulme

Not everyone likes old people—and that seems to be true in many cultures and times. Wisdom and benevolence are fine, and we certainly need grandparents, particularly if they can babysit! Yet so many people assume aging means declining competence, failing memory, lack of vitality. As well, both the good and the bad qualities imply that everyone ages the same—no room for individual variation. There's a big fuss about active old persons—but they are exceptions.

Such low expectations make life difficult for older adults. People tend to talk down to the old, especially if they show signs of age—forgetfulness, hearing problems, or impaired mobility. Older adults are especially vulnerable to such assumptions in times of transition and loss—retirement, bereavement, health problems, and major birthdays. Talking down—and talking up—send the message that people should act their age.

Students and social/health professionals in my classes and workshops on aging always ask for a list of terms to use when speaking to older adults. I initially said no, because lists assume that people are all the same. Now I end talks with my one-word rule—"Listen!" If we focus on older persons to understand who they are and what they are trying to tell us, we naturally look them in the eye, speak as we would to any adult, and let them express themselves. This book is all about listening to older adults.

We All Become Stories lets us *listen* to 12 aging voices—plus one (the author's). Ann Elizabeth Carson calls these dear friends and teachers "elders"—people who are older, but also wise and mature—like the elders in a church or in First Nations traditions. Her book offers us portraits and stories of

12 elders whom she spoke with over decades about their aging, especially the roles of memory in their later years. Very important, it also presents her voice. We can listen to her as interviewer and interpreter but also as writer reflecting on her own aging. Mary Catherine Bateson's very successful and popular *Composing a Further Life* (2010) also lets readers listen to stories of aging while they ponder their own experiences.

Carson shares with us her own changing attitudes to memory over her 40 years of chatting with older people. She started by looking at memory as something intellectual. She later learned that what and how we feel affect how we learn about the world and how we remember. Training as a psychotherapist (and as a parent!) taught her to listen carefully. She worked out an effective three-part technique:

> Ask the tough, really interesting questions.
> Listen carefully to the answer.
> Repeat the reply, but in your own words.

Do this a number of times over days, weeks, months, even years!

In each chapter, Carson gives us the background and context—how she meets the person, crucial details of his or her life and experiences, how their friendship evolves over time, and what and how she learns from their growing, deepening relationship. She also explains how she first understands something the person says and how she eventually works out his or her evolving thoughts and feelings about aging, memory, and life in general. She also presents evocative poems in each individual's story, setting a life in music and metaphor, and adding a touch of mystery. As one of her elders points out, words can only point to the memories.

Carson's poetic style makes the stories richer. For example, she describes meeting Meyer:

> *I hear Meyer before I meet him, playing piano at one of the island's evening singsongs. Hunched over the keyboard, head*

jutting forward in concentration, his long bony legs in narrow black trousers angle his knees above his waist, thrust his elbows up on either side—making his sweatered arms look like wings unfolding.

Although the interviews began long ago—some as early as four decades ago—they feel contemporary. Carson weaves in different periods, which makes the stories richer, deeper. When she started the project, she was in her late 40s; now she is in her mid-80s. Through these life stories we come to see aging as a journey—Carson often writes about walking or hiking, alone or in pairs on a trail, or together in community to view the sunset.

Even though I'm deteriorating physically, I want to break through this closing in that can come with age. I don't feel any older in my mind or my spirit; I live from day to day with whatever enjoyment is there. And when one has a sense of wonder, death is not at all a fearful thing. ~ Meyer

Carson shows us how our whole life is memory. She suggests that we ignore the usual worries about forgetting names, appointments, plans, and objects. Our memory may change and adapt as we age, and we may come to rely on what our bodies remember. One of the great revelations of this book is Carson's own admission that she started out valuing only what was "in her head" but learned to listen to her body. In *Ordinary Wisdom: Biographical Aging and the Journey of Life* (2001), Gary Kenyon and William Randall speak of "life-as-story" and "life-as-journey" to convey what Carson implies in her title *We All Become Stories*. Christina Baldwin calls her 2005 book *Storycatcher*, which term describes Carson's role here: she listens deeply so that elders can work out their own aging life story while she reflects, tells, and retells her own.

Now, because I know I remember in a sensory way I never have to say I forget. Seeing into, sensing something about what people

are really doing ... what they are feeling ... how people's emotions make meaning. That is what people remember and talk about. ~ Miriam

Ann Elizabeth Carson offers us almost a "pot of gold" at the "end of the rainbow": as we age and adapt, we may uncover talents and interests and abilities we never knew we had.

And surprisingly, as my body keeps falling apart and rotting, my painting is improving by leaps and more leaps—and it amazes me that while I can hardly work for more than 20 minutes without getting pooped, my painting is zooming, both design-wise and colour-wise, the feelings come pouring out. With every gain there's a loss and contrariwise. ~ Lev

Ellen B. Ryan, Ph.D.
Professor Emeritus
McMaster University
www.writingdownouryears.ca

Author's Introduction: A Baker's Dozen

The 12 elders who tell their stories here made extraordinary changes to find a place in a society that seldom welcome or respect old age. Their stories have changed me and inspired me, the lucky 13th, to try the same. I expected their experiences to challenge my ideas about memory and aging. What I did not anticipate, and grew to welcome and savour, was how much I learned from them and how their experiences made me more and more aware of my own aging and memory. As Meyer might say, the end of the day brings me a sense of wonder at, and gratitude for, their gifts to me.

The experiences of aging described in these pages are not universal to all cultures. The people you will meet are teachers, blue-collar workers, clerks, artists, musicians, a librarian, a housewife, and a furniture maker, all of European descent. None of them are famous; all are ordinary people looking for ways to lead satisfying lives in their old age. Seven of the storytellers are former or winter residents of New York state and Massachusetts whom I met on a remote little island off the coast of Maine, a place of lobster fishers and summer visitors. The others are city folk in Ontario: family friends and students at the seniors' centre where I taught memory strategies.

I first visited the island in the mid-1970s, on a "by chance" holiday after a conference, to relax in the peace of the place. A week of classes there in sensory awareness was my excuse for taking this extra time off. The island captured me and changed my life. A place both wild and peaceful, its trails drew me from the high rocky side down through forest to scrub, pebble beaches, and a dirt road with wooden houses weathered grey scattered here and there. I walked the two kilometres from the white clapboard schoolhouse at one end, where we had classes in the morning, past village, harbour, and fish houses, to an old shipwreck looking out to sea from a deep cove at the other end. Villagers, summer people, and visitors watched the sunset from either place, communal witness to the end of day.

Over the years, taking classes, working a stint at a local art gallery to finance a longer stay, I met year-round residents as well as summer people and made lifelong friends. Most of them were much older than I, many in their 70s and 80s, and their demeanour flew in the face of traditional ideas of 'oldness'—*in*active, forgetful, deteriorating. Falling apart. Useless.

I didn't grasp their challenge to conventional wisdom on aging at the time. The people I met were resilient and persistent, accommodating to old age in their own ways. They coped with their own and spouses' serious physical problems and fears; ever-increasing emotional, social, and economic losses; and often their communities' powerful prejudices about aging, about what they should be like, and about how they should function and remember. They seemed to accept that their life was changing, and they wondered, "How is it going to be? What do I need to do?"

These questions began to resonate for me. I returned to the island to continue studying sensory awareness, and I began to talk with Martha, Meyer, Miriam, Callum, Alice, Russell, and Lev. Martha showed me how sensory memory helped her. Callum asked me, "Why should there be words?" instead of just memory. Miriam revealed that the sensory grounded her life and memory. And Meyer observed, "Nature is my teacher now."

Why then did I live just 'in my head,' when the senses, they seemed to be saying, were the basis of everything we feel, and experience, and know. I marvelled at how Lev, despite severe illness and poverty, could wait for "the juice of life" to nourish his painting. I wondered at how 89-year-old Alice, regardless of physical and emotional travails, was able "to regiment" her energy and passion for her painting (could *I* do this?). And Russell hit home hard when he dismissed sensory memory: I suddenly saw how that attitude had hampered him—and realized that I had been doing *exactly the same thing*.

There was no avoiding sensory memory—memory we hold in the body, without thought—that shapes *all* of us, through all our lives.

Artists, musicians, teachers: was their remarkable "take" on life—so different from mine—unique? Did their close-knit island community let them make all these changes? Did it explain the profound effect their stories were having on me?

What I had learned on the island, especially about sensory awareness, encouraged me to explore further. Back home, I found five more elders to share their stories of aging and memory with me. Beatrice was my late mother's oldest friend; Emma, an older family member. I offered memory workshops at several seniors' centres in Toronto, and there I met Avram, Rebecca, and Rivka.

As we came to know each other, I realized both their fear of mental decline and their desire for independence. They seemed to expect intellectual deterioration with old age, even though only illness, stress, and medication seemed to affect their memory. They felt increasing need to belong in a community, but it demanded they act "old"—dependent, confused, inactive—and this threatened their fierce desire for independence.

To earn acceptance and a sense of belonging, they had to live with traditional stereotypes of oldness all around them. Yet, as we see below, they constantly challenged and refuted these beliefs, thus expanding their—and our—notions of what aging and old age can be. They navigated the Scylla and Charybdis of these apparent paradoxes with the consummate skill of people who had been making changes and difficult choices throughout their long, often challenging lives. Now they had to create places for themselves in a youth-obsessed society. As they became more frail, they faced enormous adjustments, but they could indeed adapt and live "as well as possible ... so that 'feeling good is enough'" (Miriam's words).

Those like Rivka and Avram who had floundered and been in danger of "sinking into deep days of depression," as

Emma put it, needed very little encouragement to reassemble lives that had fallen apart under the pressure of poverty and unremitting hard work or fear of the future. They renewed old passions and found new interests. Like the others, they knew that cultivating a continuing passion or some other way to give meaning and value to life makes pain and loss tolerable. Sometimes allowing loss to deepen, learning "to let it walk beside you" as Martha did, can bring unexpected strength, as Beatrice and Emma found, and I have too.

To fly in the face of conventional wisdom about aging and memory requires enormous resolve and strength. Where do these restorative powers come from? It is almost as if life offers people the proverbial pot of gold at the end of the rainbow—just when they need it. But the pot has been there all along: the recipients, perhaps unawares, have been filling it with the experiences of a lifetime.

Reflecting on my own beliefs and fears and my unconscious absorption of the stereotypes that I was questioning, I see how my questions and discoveries have transformed my life. Aging and old age cast a spotlight on the reality of human frailty and vulnerability at every life stage, and they reveal that "aging" is not just something that "happens" to the old, but can be a process of self-integration, a lifelong evolution relevant to all ages.

The people whose stories you read below had no illusions. Life, aging, and old age are tough: "a tall order" as Meyer said, more difficult for people who are poor, gravely ill, or not used to "looking within." And a lot easier within a supportive community as Martha knew, Rivka discovered, Russell grudgingly accepted, and I am now realizing with gratitude.

But no one tells you when you are young that life can remain interesting and worthwhile when you are old, even become *more* interesting and worthwhile. Old age is your last hurrah—not only a challenge but a privilege, even a joy, not available when you are young. You can call on and value resources you have developed over a lifetime, discover interests and talents you never knew you had, cultivate latent sources of strength and resolve, and create new ways to take pleasure in life.

I was in my late 40s, and they were from 75 to 83, when I first met these elders and talked with them about being old and about memory. The more I listened and learned, the more I realized how our views and experiences of memory help us adapt to the changing circumstances and abilities of our old age. And the more I wanted to write their stories, to give a voice—one we seldom hear—to ordinary people's experiences of what it is like to be old.

As you and I explore these elders' stories of being old and of memory, our journey will open up a world of oldness people rarely speak of. We see too the vast and rich domain of sensory memory, which neither they nor I "had ever thought of in that way, as memory," as Alice observed. Each of their stories can, in its own way, open our eyes if we have always thought that memory is 'in our heads,' separate from our bodies, our social relationships, and our environments.

It is my hope that *We All Become Stories* will appeal to your curiosity about aging and about memory. You can truly welcome old age when you learn about it from people you have come to know and value.

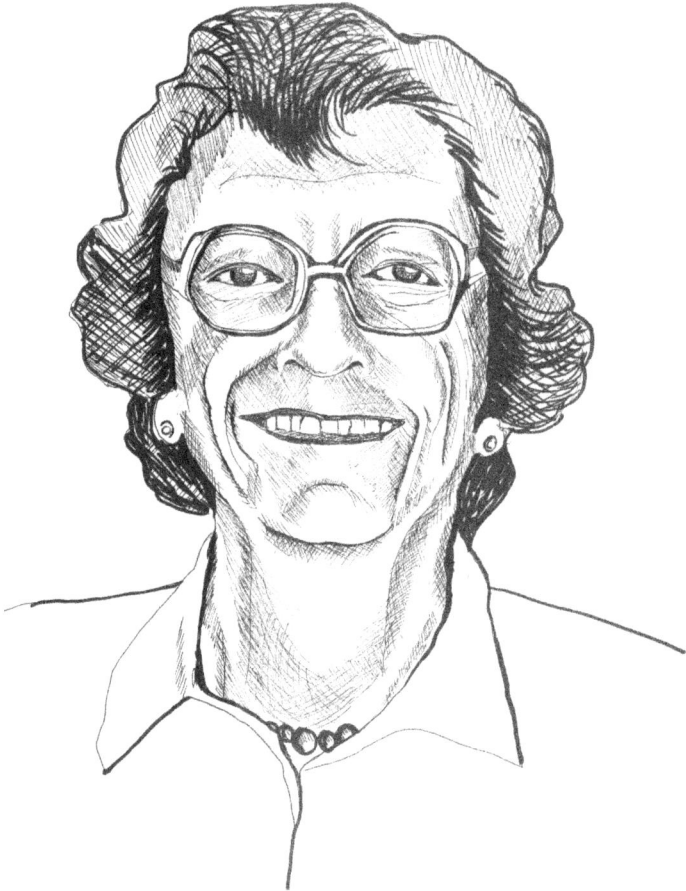

Martha

Life's Work: Martha's Story

"Now I understand why I did certain things. I can accept more … All you have to do is catch hold of the tail and pull it … reaching back for the spirit that was there."

Catching Up

There is an island an hour and a half by ferry from the Maine shore, named by native people long years ago, marked by Columbus on his navigation charts. Year-round residents fish lobster in winter, now a few cod in summer, and whatever they catch in winter. Broiled, steamed, or in cream sauce if it's a day old, this is what you eat, if you want fish. Take your pick. It's not to everyone's taste, this island: no cars—except for emergency services and trucks for hauling traps in winter, luggage in summer. Messages to the mainland used to pass through the coast guard on the smaller island that creates the protected harbour. Now there is electricity in year-round homes, the coast guard has been automated, and there are more than three phones. The lighthouse no longer needs a keeper, the foghorn is timed and sometimes does not know when to shut off, booming in sunshine, reminding of storms and ships seeking harbour.

Whenever I reach the island I watch for her as the ferry nears the dock at low tide. I see her standing on the pier, high above the water, silhouetted against the old inn, from whose third-floor windows she looks out to sea on rainy days. Short, slight, dressed usually in red and blue, with salt-and-pepper hair moistly curling in the early morning mist under her round-brimmed white hat, she smiles broadly as we draw closer. Conversation on shore and aboard the boat stops in anticipation of landing, and I hear her soft, southern drawl: "I thought this day would never come."

Up the steep gangplank, I am finally ashore, a little unsteady after an hour and a half on rough water. She gestures to me to make sure my luggage is on the truck to the hostel for my two-week stay. We hug, lightly. It has been a while, but lightly is enough for old bones. We walk up the dusty hill to the inn together, touch hands, smiling, bodies leaning towards each others'. How could there be words? I know she has planned a day for us to walk and talk.

"Is lobster bisque and lobster roll being too much of a glutton?" I ask.

"Have what you want. I always do on my first day. I never can resist the Indian pudding."

Lunch at the inn, where Martha is staying, is catch-up time since our last phone call—families, recent happenings, and a brief health report. This time Martha tells me, "Well, I'm not as steady on the trails as I used to be."

"And I still can't walk for too long. That old back accident lingers on, so I'll steady you on the rough bits if you don't mind if we don't go too far?"

"That's just fine. I don't think I'm up to much more than you are. You need to pace yourself when you first get here."

We sit for a while after lunch in the rocking chairs on the inn's narrow porch, watch passengers board the ferry heading back to the mainland. Then, with fewer hikers on the trails, we set off, winding through the woods to the rocky coast on the other side of the island. It was on this trail that we had had our first long conversation and begun a lifelong friendship.

Martha and I had met on the island in 1975 at a sensory awareness workshop. The work is almost completely non-verbal—learning through experiencing something, being touched or moved by it, rather than thinking about it—"An exercise in faithfulness." Classes in the morning, a quiet, solitary lunch to absorb the morning's new awareness, and then exploring the island.

It's very small, just over three kilometres long and one and a half kilometres wide, a high rocky shore on one side, on the low side a small village around a fisherman's harbour protected by the even-smaller island. Private and state conservancies protect much of the island from development, making it an ideal place to wander undisturbed for hours. When you encounter people on the trails—artists making for a quiet spot, hikers circumnavigating the coastal trails—they too "are not much for conversation," as Martha says.

We both treasure silence, stopping, wordless, to look at a newly blooming flower or the sun streaking through the evergreens and turning the pine needles a russet-gold. Martha is a knowledgeable birdwatcher and takes a scientist's pleasure in naming them and the rare wildflowers everywhere in such abundance. We arrive at our chosen place on the coast, sit on the rocks breathing the salty air and pine scent, watching the ships on the rounded horizon sailing for larger ports, the nesting gulls, and sometimes a school of dolphins or a pair of migrating whales. And then, as usual, we talk.

Growing Up, Marriage, Tragedy

Over the years I learned that Martha grew up on the edge of a small town in the American southwest, the third of four children of prosperous, middle-class folks. They were fundamentalist Christians rearing their offspring in fear of God's punishment and guilt for earthly sins, and in unquestioning obedience to their parents.

Martha said, "When I professed my faith in Christ as a little girl I am sure it was more from fear of hell and damnation than it was the love of the Lord, not the kind of personal relationship with God that I have now." Although she knew her father was a good man, he was very strict with her when she was past being his "little pet." She couldn't see then that "his strictness and his faith were the way he had of loving me. I counted on his strength later on, when my life was so painful."

Her mother was a hard worker, "not so much with feelings; I don't think I ever remember her in that way. She always wanted to get her work done … didn't have time to talk. When you did something that displeased her she'd withdraw and get silent. That's hard for a child. And my father said, 'Mind your mother and don't talk back' … see … my thing was I didn't express myself, and Laura, my older sister always did."
She felt her sisters always told her what to do, as if she didn't know anything, and they never wanted her with them. "I can see why, now I've had my own children, but it hurt me then. My mother never took up for me on that.

"And James [her brother]. Well! He was the little prince! He was awful sick when he was a little boy and almost died. Everybody thought he would, and I remember I was six years old but my father took me in to say goodbye. I felt *so sick* that morning, and Leila, who had come to help, laid me across the kitchen chair on my stomach. And I felt guilty too. I never knew why until years later when I started to work through some of those feelings, how I resented him. Here he was dying, and I'm sure I felt responsible."

Martha felt isolated from her peers and thought of herself as an introvert. She and her siblings were "supposed to be an example to others"—no movies, dancing, or playing cards. So she read a lot, and that's how she learned to excel— an escape from social pressure. She went to college, majored in chemistry, and worked as a technician until she married and had her two boys three years apart. "It was all we thought we ever wanted," she said, "and I married a man who could absolutely charm you … See, I think I was a dependent person. I was still crying about what my father said, and I rebelled and got married. But I apparently still wanted somebody to tell me what to do, and G. was very good at it. I also had feelings that somehow I was responsible for everything that happened. If anything went wrong I'd feel this tightness in my neck and sometimes a pain, right here, between my shoulder blades, thinking it was more or less my fault. G. assured me it was. He kept himself very aloof ... I had this closed-out feeling all the time that I used to get. So there was a void in my life."

In her middle years Martha suffered the loss of everything that had ever had any meaning for her. Her two sons died—the older one, first, from pancreatic cancer in early adulthood. The younger one committed suicide in adolescence only three years later. Both of her parents had died. She and her husband divorced a few years later because "G. would never talk about the boys, and I knew I had to. I remember my friend Bonnie saying: 'Martha, we have always talked about Frank, and we're not going to stop.' I was so grateful to her; I knew I needed to talk. How else could I keep on remembering him? How could anyone? G. just wouldn't, he'd always been cold and distant, and now I knew I couldn't live with that anymore."

A New Life
A New Calling

I met Martha in 1975, 10 years after the suicide of her second son, and she was still struggling to find purpose and meaning "now and for the future." My own marriage, and family life as I had always envisaged it, had just ended. But I was acutely aware—almost embarrassed—that unlike her I still had four children to bring up, although I certainly had never thought I would be doing it alone. That summer she and I walked the trails, getting to know each other, sharing our delight in the island's bounty and in the insights that Claudia's classes awakened. Eventually we were able to acknowledge—to ourselves and to each other—how adrift, confused, and frightened we felt.

We talked on the phone during the winter about the ways we were exploring the next steps in our lives, both reading Jung, and Gestalt psychology. One night she sounded especially excited:

"Oh, Ann. I know what the Lord wants me to do."

"What's that, Martha?"

"He wants me to be a good friend."

"But you *already* are a good friend."

"Yes. Maybe. But that's not what He means. He wants me to befriend other people in trouble."

"How are you going to do that?"

"I've enrolled in a course in pastoral counselling!"

She wrote to tell me how much our conversations had helped her, which surprised me. I had felt so supported by her, and somewhat shamefaced, because it seemed to me that her losses were much greater than mine. We both decided to enrol in Claudia's class the next summer, and when we met it was wonderful to hear her say, "What I'm learning about myself—I just can't believe how things have opened up for me."

Over the next three weeks, as we walk old trails and explore new ones, Martha slowly unravels for me what she has been learning during the past winter. For many years she has been engaged in a journey of self-discovery. Now, she is delving more deeply, discovering new layers of what her life had been, so that she "can put the pieces together and find meaning" for her life "as it has been, and for the future."

"Putting the puzzle together, where there's a missing piece," I ask, "would you then go and talk about that with someone to get the waters ruffled … get things going?"

"Well, I could do that, or I would just start talking to the missing piece."

"An internal dialogue?"

"As Robert Johnson [psychologist and author] says, all you have to do is catch hold of the tail and pull it."

"What else do you do?"

"Dreams. Active imagination. Paying attention to my body, like the tense feeling I get in my neck. My journal every day. In conversation with someone. When something sparks, you kind of pick it up, maybe then, maybe later. That goes back to the painful part."

"Trying to put it away. Because of the pain?"

"Yes."

"You never really do?" I ask.

"No. I don't think you do. Even when you want to ignore it, you can't give your body away, or those deep feelings."

"What about the joyful parts? Do they get put away?"

"Yes," she said. "See, what I did, growing up and in my marriage, was sit on all my feelings. But when I let myself pay attention, as the painful ones came out, the joyful ones came back too, and you see things that you didn't see before. Like right now, talking to you about this, I remember all the times we've laughed and cried walking the trails and talking ... The telephone can be a lifeline, can't it?"

"It certainly has been for me," I reply.

Breaking Through—Reaching Back

Unhappiness in her marriage had first alerted Martha to how distanced she was from her feelings. The deeper she probed into the conflicts of the marriage, the scarier it became. When her friend Bonnie reminded her that "God has not given us the spirit of fear but the power of love and a sound mind," all the scriptures she heard as a child, "the songs and all that—just came pouring into me. It was really wonderful ... and I had forgotten them."

God's love broke through all the guilt and fear when she realized that she could "look more to the loving God in the scriptures that was there all along. I was His child and worthy of His love." She was starting to feel God's love through other people who "weren't brought up in that same strictness." It changed her life. "I can look back now and feel so sorry for that little girl."

For Martha, to be "opened up" in this way meant that she became aware of deeper layers of emotions and physical sensations and then of the memories that came with them.

"I was unhappy enough that I knew I had to ... One time over a rather trivial thing I blew my stack with G. 'I hate you.' I literally went to pieces. That was the first time I was ever angry. I felt guilty about it. Then I started looking at myself—this quiet, agreeable, presumably loving person ... and then the shadow side, all the turmoil inside ... ugly, negative things all bottled up. I was a *divided* person. I saw that *ever since then* I've been trying to integrate that shadow side. As I do, I become more of what I was pretending to be. Isn't that wonderful! I'm not as much of a hypocrite. That's true, isn't it?"

"That's really true."

"The amazing thing is how blind I was to those feelings that were within me all the time because I was denying them. I really think I was numb. I remember Bonnie talking to me: 'Why aren't you angry? That would make me so mad.' I couldn't allow myself. I wasn't *feeling* angry one bit. I was detached from myself."

"And you had good models for that. As you thawed ..."

"'As I thawed' is right!"

"Then you could allow yourself to feel what you'd put away?"

"Hmm. Some of it. Some of the feelings were pretty violent. I'm sure there's a lot in me that hasn't come out yet. Maybe I don't want them! But I'm working on that. You do learn how to dissipate it in ways that don't hurt yourself and won't hurt other people."

During a trip to Europe, the first without her husband, she realized that she had felt like a person with her friends, not an object, as G. treated her, as if she was someone interesting in her own right. She came back and told G. how she felt feminine and good about herself for the first time ... and he said he should never have let her go on the trip.

She went into therapy because of not being valued in her marriage and feeling swamped by all her emotions: anger, fear of the anger, guilt about being angry, and the painful physical accompaniments like stomach, neck and head aches—Martha eventually called them "warnings." The psychiatrist's telling her that her anger was the best thing that ever happened to her spurred her to start looking inside herself, to what her body was trying to tell her, and to begin to understand more of her feelings. Her husband "kept after" her, so she quit therapy after three sessions. After her son became ill, they went as a family. She didn't know if it was helpful to the others, but it was for her. She found out that she wasn't crazy, that everything wasn't her fault, that she was sitting there like a sponge soaking up everything that was thrown at her. She knew that it was time for her to put her feet on the ground and become an independent person.

Beneath the numbness and the anger she found early feelings of rejection, of feeling unworthy and not valued as she grew up, and sometimes where they came from, "like writing for my birth certificate for the first time, and it was made out in my brother John's name. By then my parents were dead, and so I didn't know how that happened, although I assumed they must have wanted a boy. I didn't like it at all, it made me feel real low. I know I felt responsible for him for a long time, from the stories I remember."

As adults she and her brother went on family camping trips together, and she saw him as a hard-working man, not a spoiled child. Later, when he was helping her through her divorce, he apologized for not realizing all she had gone through, and Martha felt acknowledged at last.

When he became seriously ill, she realized that the guilt had dissipated and she "feels gratitude for him and fear of losing him, at the same time." She knew now, having been through the loss of sons, husband, and parents, that she must "release him and free myself from the compulsion to care."

"That sounds like a kind of forgetting, Martha."

"Well, I suppose it is, 'cause when I release all that responsibility I can forget about that and care about him the way I want to now, as a friend."

Working through the feelings that clustered around her sense of responsibility, she found other feelings surfacing—"like I'm beginning to understand my mother more, how she must have felt. There she was, far from home, in a strange place homesteading. And she was the oldest child, with that kind of responsibility to begin with, and then the constant work and her not feeling valued—I can relate to that … the kind of caring a child doesn't notice as care until you grow up and start to do it yourself—and with about as much thanks."

"But you know, I still identify more with my father. He and I were both helpers … Dad would help mother with the laundry, things like that. He instructed us to do what mother wanted and to help her. I expected the same thing in my marriage and was surprised when I didn't get it—G. wasn't the helping kind."

She carried her father's injunction to care for others with her, as well as his strong faith in God, but from a different perspective—"not fear, but the power of love."

Opening Up to the World
The Importance of Community

Martha says that when her feelings swamp her and memories come up, or when she is wondering what to do, she needs someone to talk to. "You get another perspective, so you don't have to carry the load all by yourself. It's much harder to find any meaning when you can't share what is happening with someone."

Her friend Bonnie was a godsend. A neighbour when they both first married, they became good friends, "so she has a lot of the same memories. Sometimes she reminds me of things I've forgotten—probably wanted to forget. She's been wonderful, can see the feelings in me I can get separated from. I mean, like we're talking now isn't social chatter. It isn't everyone you can share with."

"No, not like we do, no," I replied. "And it seems you need a lot of time, to be able to take it all in, find out where it fits, how it's affected your life, what you might want to change."

"That's right, you do. It's a lot, isn't it? But see, we're talking about painful memories; there are wonderful memories that carry all the way through as well. In the same way a feeling of joy will come up, and you can share that. I think you remember what you share in a different way than when you don't.

"Like Grethe [an island resident] is reliving memories every day at the inn, talking about growing up on the island. As you get older there's no one left who shared your life, and you must learn to tell your story. She does it so well. If she didn't, no one would listen, and she couldn't share anything. Her memories would fade."

Martha's friends and church community became integral to her life. When her first son died, she recognized that people were not only basic to her well-being and growth, but to her very survival, because God's love—"which was not much in my childhood"—came to her through them.

When her second son died, Martha's neighbours and her therapist were at her side at the hospital. Her husband wanted them to go home, but Martha told him: "I can't stand it if I don't have people. With that, N. [her therapist] got up and left. She knew I was all right, told me 'You aren't consciously feeling it but I look at your family, I see that you are the strong one, you had more background and love growing up than your husband did.' God's love coming to me from other people helped me get through it. All my family were busy with their own lives."

The struggle to hear God's love through other competing conversations is lifelong for Martha. She knows that she will always have to keep dealing with the fear and grief instilled in childhood. But it's not what she wants to focus on now. In the aftermath of overwhelming tragedy, when it is so easy for doubt to creep in, she needs people who believe in God's love—who are a means of His love, as she has made up her mind she will be—to remind her not to forget that she too is "His child and worthy of love."

A Good Friend

In the years that followed I experienced what it was like to be Martha's "good friend," as well as her longtime friend. When my younger son took his own life, she knew immediately what I was going through, what to say, what to do. She knew that my "family was busy with their own lives"—and their own mourning—and how alone I was.

It was becoming harder for her to travel, but she came up to Canada the three following autumns. We explored lakes in Muskoka and Georgian Bay, not talking much, although she urged me to find people I could talk to, well aware that she couldn't be the only one.

One time I asked her, "How did you do this, Martha? How did you get to where you are now?"

"Eventually you learn to let it walk beside you," she replied—words I carry with me always.

When I would thank her for being there, for being my rock, she always replied, "But it's the Lord's spirit within me, not just me, it's God's love coming through."

"He chose a wonderful vessel."

"I think it's the willingness to be used."

"For that ... and nothing else? You've not allowed yourself to be used in ways that you don't agree with. And that's hard."

"Oh, it's because I hadn't really stood for myself ... Now it just means that I plan to stand up for pretty much what I believe."

"You've come a long way."

"Yes, but I was the first one in the family who went through difficulties. Until it hit the rest of them, they didn't know. You will get through this, Ann. I know you're not feeling that way right now, but you're strong. And I pray for you every day."

After a five-year absence from the Island, Martha knew I needed to come back and surprised me with a two-week holiday there for my 70th birthday at a hostel close to where she stayed. Smelling the hedge roses, lying on the rocks in the mist, my whole body loosened as I sank into the island's sensuous embrace. As I remembered the companionship and happiness in all the familiar places I felt as if I might be able to let my son's absence "walk beside me." For years I had thought I would never write again, but here, aware once more of the "open present," something "opened up" for me, and I began to write poetry once more.

Setting Priorities

Martha was having her own struggle. She needed to resolve the conflict between "being used as a channel of love" and being "used up" by the needs of those for whom she is a "good friend," whether family, friends, or people in her pastoral care. The more she worked through her feelings to understand where they came from, and the blocks that had prevented her from remembering them, the more intense the process became in every way—physical, emotional, and mental. She needed more solitude to reflect, to work through dreams and inner conversations, to think about what was happening in her life, and to journal. She disliked being too busy and wondered "how people who stay so busy, how they're able to do it. Now I know at home I can't do as much as I used to do. I can go a certain amount of time, and then I want to stay home and be quiet."

"You're saying 'quiet,' not, 'take a rest.'"

"No. I don't take a nap."

"I wonder whether, if you take into account the amount of remembering and thinking and integrating everything that you do in a day, that you would actually say that you don't do as much."

"No. It's life's work. See, I'm internal. I mean I was always internal, but it's being internal in a different way. Integration, rather than just carrying on conversations with yourself."

"So, it sounds as if you may be slowing down physically, but sort of speeding up mentally?"

"That's right! That's really true."

"Are you getting tired?"

"No, I'm all right. This is kind of hard, what we're talking about, isn't it."

"Yes, it is. But it's good to talk about it, not just hold it all inside."

"You need that too, Ann."

"I know it, Martha; I get so much of that with you …"

"Lifelines," we smiled.

Martha loved the island and invited most of her family and many friends to visit her while she was there. Gradually friends and family take over her place of quiet retreat and regeneration, planning their visits to coincide with hers—a unique opportunity to be with her—as indeed I have two years later.

She had missed the intervening summer to recuperate from major surgery, and this summer she was looking forward especially to rest and recuperation, but it hasn't happened. By the time I arrive she is close to the end of her stay, and feeling overwhelmed. She has been "too much with people," is expecting another group, and is panicky about how little time she has left.

Sitting on the inn's verandah after my first-day lunch, she let me know, kindly but firmly, that we cannot plan any walks or dinners together, that we will just have to "go with the flow and meet by chance." I was heavy with disappointment, and, to my surprise, with anger. I had come a long distance, under difficult physical circumstance, to be with her. We had planned the time, and timing, together. I struggled with feelings of rejection, and of being unacknowledged.

But as her friend I could hardly quarrel with her need to care for herself. We had often talked about how hard it was to put ourselves first, not last, as we had been raised to do. Now she was "going against the grain." While not liking the consequences, I could only applaud her strategy, and, given our love for each other and how well she knew me, the courage it must take to stick to her resolve. And do a little "working through" myself.

Aging Equals Memory Loss?

Finally, we do "meet by chance" at the inn after dinner and walk along the gentle path to the bench at Ice Pond. The placid ducks ignore us, forage among the high reeds, occasionally scolding an errant young one. Gulls call, swooping in and out for a freshwater bath.

"It's hard for me to be distant from you, Ann, and I know it's been hard for you, but I really had to do some thinking. See, something has been worrying me, and I needed to work it through before we talked. We're sometimes pretty intense together aren't we?"

"For sure, we certainly can be."

"There seems to be more to be intense about."

"Do you remember Florida Scott-Maxwell writing about that?"

"Yes, but not exactly what she said."

"She said: 'My heart must be a miracle of quiet to endure the intensity of my life.'"

"I need a lot of quiet."

"I know Martha. I do too. It's hard when needing the quiet and seeing each other collide. You know I miss you."

"I know it! And I miss you too. Now I'd like to tell you something, if that's OK."

"Of course. I'm all ears."

She's been having a little difficulty with short-term memory. She hates it when she can't remember names but doesn't put that down to age—she's never been good at absorbing a name, noting (correctly), "If you don't store it in your memory bank, it isn't going to be there for you to pull out."

She remembers how people look, especially their eyes, the way they move, and how they talk, not just what they talk about. And then their connections to other people she knows, and where they come from, places they've been. But to her a name is just a name; it doesn't have the same kinds of associations that relationships do.

I tell her that's the way I remember too—focusing on faces and places—but that names are more like labels for me.

"Oh, good, that makes me feel better; a label isn't the person, is it? I don't think forgetting appointments is so bad; I put it down to not looking in my appointment book. What I do is I just release it. If it doesn't come, I release it, and it comes."

"That seems to work for a lot of people. You talked about releasing feelings too ... Is it the same sort of thing?"

"Somewhat, like I forget about it. But I don't want the old feelings to come back, like I do other things! Right now, what I'm more concerned about is going into a room and forgetting what I came for, especially when I've been too busy."

She knows it's mostly how you handle it, not old age and she's read that older people can learn new things and remember them as well as young people—"some things better, like history and so forth. But my recall is slower than it was."

"You know, Martha, that's pretty amazing, because that is one of the age-related forms of memory loss that has been well documented. And you are observing that for yourself."

"So, that *is* aging?"

"Yes, but most other memory loss is due to certain medications, to illness, and to stress, and older people have a lot of stress."

Martha agrees; the loss of friends, family, even moving from her home of 48 years took a lot out of her. But now that she is older, she's not as physically active. It isn't just a slowing down of recall: her whole body is slow. She accomplishes much less because she moves more slowly and tires more rapidly. This bothers her—the way she aches in the morning and forgets things, because physically she wants to feel like she used to, walking the rocky trails on her own. "To just bound out of bed in the morning would be wonderful."

"It certainly would! Physical stress—it's hard to take, it's like a loss of parts of your body."

"I'll say. It *is*, you know, and sometimes you don't know yourself at all! And now I'm going to tell you one [loss], but there's a problem because of an emotional thing I haven't worked out yet."

She will put away jewellery or money, something of value, and then forget where she's put it. Then she'll start looking back on who was in the house and think that maybe they took it, which she feels is an unworthy thought. It bothers her, and she doesn't know where it comes from.

"It doesn't occur to you to say, 'Now I must have forgotten where I put that'?"

"See, that's the step I'm missing, right there."

I tell her that many people in my workshops on memory and aging often "forget" to do their homework, and about one woman who said that it was because if she made a mistake she didn't want to look stupid. I ask her if she doesn't want to be seen as someone who forgets, and she says yes, that's it. Then I ask her what would be so awful about that, adding that I forget, my daughter forgets, my granddaughter forgets. "Is it that you think only old people forget?" She agrees—even though she "knows better," knows that forgetting happens at any age; when she forgets *now* she can't help thinking "going downhill physically means you're bound to forget."

"I make the same kind of association, Martha, between forgetting and my aches and pains. But I can't put it down to age; it's because I've been so sick, and that's stressful, makes me forget."

"So you think we connect getting older with being feeble, and connect feebleness with being mentally incompetent?" Martha asks. "Not being able to control one's body is very threatening, but not nearly as threatening as being mentally incapacitated."

"You know people keep saying about getting old, 'She's still as sharp as a tack,' as if that's a surprise. But we all know a lot of older people who are very sharp, and younger ones who aren't. You said so yourself, and you've told me that you've read that older people can remember just as well as younger ones. And yet, blanking out when you get older seems to carry with it the threat of 'my mind is turning to mush, I'm getting older.' I think the idea that forgetting is *always* because you're old is an ageist stereotype."

"That instead of thinking that way we really should be feeding ourselves the other: 'I may be having a temporary lapse.'"

"Right! You've not lost something, you've misplaced it. But you haven't misplaced your *mind*."

Putting It All Together

It was another two years before Martha and I met on the island again, in 2002. Family stayed with her, friends came and went at other accommodations. She had developed an inner-ear problem and had several scary falls.

"I can feel myself going and can't prevent it; I fall backwards and can't right myself. I haven't broken any bones, which at my age is pretty good, but the girls don't want me to walk by myself."

I was staying nearby again and could use the house phone. We talked every day ("like we used to"). Some days, if she felt like it, we walked along the flatter, less demanding lower coast road along the shore—she with her striders, I with my cane.

"Well," said Martha, when we stopped to rest on a rock, "I said I'd tell you how it turned out when I forgot something. I don't blame people any more when I forget where I've put something, and I'm glad—I know I've put it someplace. But I still don't like anyone *else* to think I'm forgetful! I've been working on that."

She and a friend attend a regular meeting, and Martha will offer to drive her and then sometimes forget to do so. The friend asked her if she was becoming forgetful, and Martha had "a furious headache." After thinking and journaling about it for a while, she realized that she was feeling too responsible for her friend. She discussed this with her and the friend agreed to ask when she wanted a lift and that Martha could say no. "I probably wouldn't, but it was nice to know I could."

Her anger surprised her; she thought at first that it was about aging and forgetting and then realized that "something had been hooked—I had that tight feeling in my neck." She thought through why she was forgetting and realized that she was angry about being taken for granted—"just like I was when I was growing up, and by G." Like her mother, she withdraws, goes inside, and suppresses her anger about the years of being taken for granted. And gets angry with her friend instead for insinuating that she's forgetful.

I ask her which comes first—understanding (and peace) and then more memories or memories and then understanding?

"Well," she replies, "you start with an ache or a pain, like my headache, then the feelings. You can put it off if there's too much pain to handle right then—but then, when you see that the selves are integrating ... because of what you're doing we're calling it memories, but really they are *pieces of one's life*, and so you become more of a whole person as you do this."

"So, with your friend and driving to the meeting, you felt the tail, grabbed it, and gave it a pull."

"I *did!* But see, there's another tail I can't quite find to take hold on."

"What's that?"

Family Stories and Stereotypes

"Well, it's seems silly. I don't walk every day like I used to—it made me feel good but now I want the time for other things; I can't imagine a day without my journal." She knows that a healthy body and a healthy mind go together, but she just doesn't want to pay much attention to her body anymore because it reminds her of all the aches and pains and she's afraid her mind will go downhill with her body.

She'd mentioned how a sick stomach, a headache or a sore neck alerts her to something that she's forgotten or that needs looking at. "Now you're saying that if you pay attention to those aches and pains, then you have to think your mind is going ... that you won't be able to remember, or to work through the memories and the feelings and understand your life. That's a puzzle, a bit of a contradiction."

"That's it! See, it's that I don't want to think I'll forget more and more as I get older. Growing up, we were never so much with our bodies. A sound mind was always more important than a sound body—that was taken for granted. I know there's a difference in the kinds of pains, but I can't seem to separate out the twinges that tell me to pay attention to what I'm feeling, from my body aching because it's wearing out, from thinking that getting old means my mind won't work as well."

"You can't see which tail to grab."

"No! And I don't want to get discouraged."

"Martha, are you thinking you won't find God's love coming through if you forget more?"

"Maybe that's it."

"You've said that you discovered 'the spirit that was always in you,' and 'it's not just me, it's God's love coming through me.' How could that change?"

"This is a whole other level of trust, isn't it? I guess that's what I'll be working on. I knew there'd be something."

"There's the tail!"

"I know it!"

Full Circle with Martha

Walking on the island ...
Years along the lower coast road, a bell buoy
carries our words in the wind.
Yew berries wrinkle our noses on the way
to Ice Pond—ducks decoy silent. Up over
grey crags to peer into the gull rookery ...

In between ...
Dust devils bowling along the road
to the horse farm in Oklahoma, an Alaska
glacier—
helicopter barely makes it out ahead of the
storm.
Algonquin, Muskoka, Haliburton fires by the
lake at night.
Diving from a boat in Georgian Bay, drying on
the silky quartz
of Fox Islands. A three-day, six-restaurant tour
of Toronto—
well, you wanted multicultural!

And always back to the island ...
Getting lost near Smiley's Cove, waist high
in mud and reeds, guided by
your friend's voice to the sea.
Sitting on the church steps drinking in warm
roses,
meadow smells, Casals' cello.
Huddled high on the fire escape freeze-
wrapped
in blankets the night the Northern Lights
sang—
making that wonderful music.

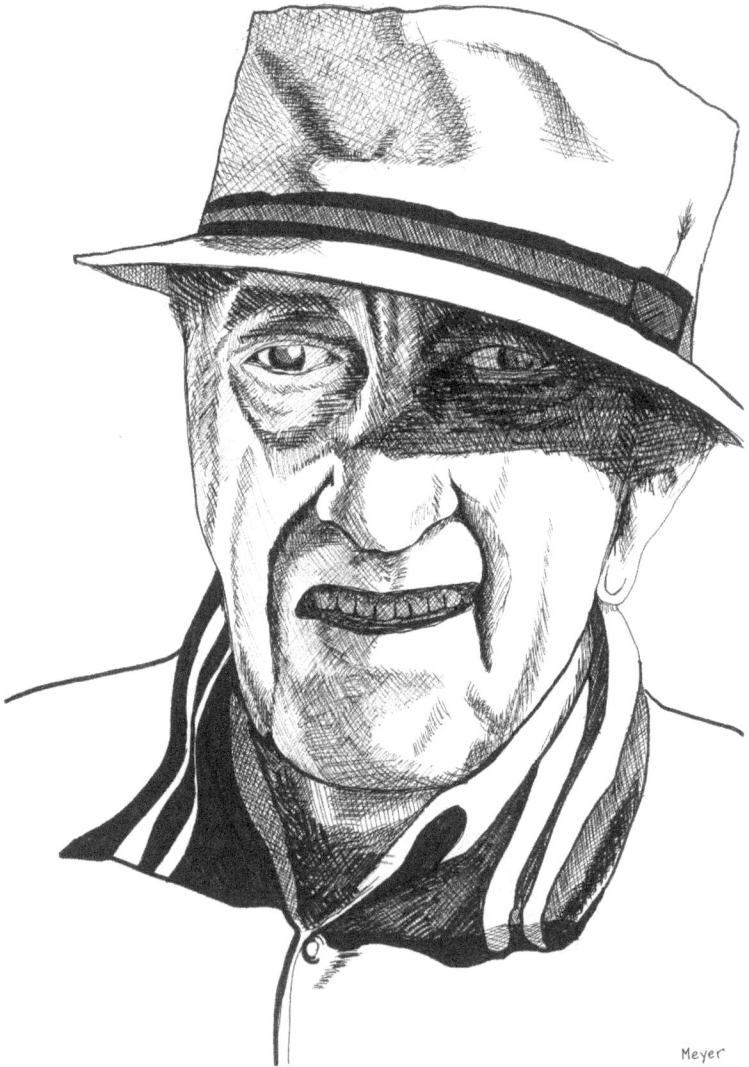

Meyer

Making Sense of the World: Meyer's Story

"Are you learning something? Nature is my teacher now."

I hear Meyer before I meet him, playing piano at one of the island's evening singsongs. Hunched over the keyboard, head jutting forward in concentration, his long bony legs in narrow black trousers angle his knees above his waist, thrust his elbows up on either side—making his sweatered arms look like wings unfolding. He shoots a quick, quizzical glance over his shoulder as his fingers ripple a change in the music from his own composition to one that the audience, sitting in chairs or cushions around the fire, can sing. A woman's rich contralto picks up the melody, leading until we find it, all singing together. Meyer grins, the tempo picks up, and his feet, one on the pedal, the other on the floor, thump out the changing rhythm as one song flows into another.

Long-time Islanders

Meyer and his wife, Miriam, are New Yorkers born and bred, both the children of Jewish immigrants from Austria in the early 20th century. They had taken evening classes in sensory awareness in New York and travelled to the island for two-week intensives. After they retired, they spent their summers there, and over the years they became island institutions.

Whether you set out to hike the trails, go to classes, walk to and from the general store and post office or to the harbour at the other end of the island, you pass their cottage nestled in a small, treed meadow at the hub of it all.

In good weather, you'll glimpse them through the wild rose hedge having morning coffee or afternoon tea on the porch. And you can be sure that if you walk by regularly they'll notice you before too long. I often meet Meyer on the island's only road—tall, gangly, sporting a pork-pie hat over a fringe of grey hair. He wears a leg brace and walks with a cane, limping a little, a shopping bag in his other hand, looking around as if he were seeing the houses and gardens for the first time. More often he'll be talking intently to someone, bag on the side of the dirt road, gesticulating with his free hand. Meyer "certainly has a way with him," Miriam says, adding that it's a good thing he does, because once he starts talking he's like the ancient mariner in Coleridge's poem who fixes you with his glittering eye so that it's hard to "get a word in edgeways."

It's true. Meyer can dominate a conversation, and at first I found him overbearing and even pompous at times. But I'm soon drawn in as he talks with his friends about music, world affairs, literature, the island's history, and its rare orchids and birds, moving knowledgeably from one subject to the next with awesome ease.

Though always attentive to my well-being and interested in my ideas, Meyer rarely shares personal details and usually downplays emotions as dangerous distractions from the pursuit of "understanding." It is his passion for music, sensory awareness (now a particular interest of mine), and making sense of our lives that betrays him as caring deeply, not only for his friends and family but also for humankind and the "state of the world."

He has survived the Great Depression and a "sparse" childhood, the horrors of a world war, an unpredictable profession, and the discipline of lifelong frugality, so that he and Miriam can live "well enough" in old age. Now he copes daily not only with painful physical infirmity—which he shrugs off as "coming with the territory" of age—but also with deafness, which robs him of fully enjoying music. This loss has led him to focus on "what makes sense of it all" and eventually to discover a deeper connection to the sensory, in nature and within himself.

The Languages of Music and Art

The following summer Miriam invited me for dinner one night and showed me how to cook the best scallops I ever ate. Afterwards, she sits back smiling as Meyer "holds forth," and I "give as good as I get."

Having heard him play the piano, I want to know more about his music. He says that music has always been a natural part of his life. His father was a singer, and Meyer started playing piano at five or six and was found to have perfect pitch. Skimming over the personal, Meyer adds that he thinks people like himself who "get into some kind of art do so because it was a sensory part of their life very early on—in their family or school or community.

"And it follows from there," Meyer says. "Over the years, I've come to think that the arts may take this shape or that—a sonata, a painting, a poem—but what they have in common is that they all come through the senses before taking a particular form. Mine comes to me through my ears. Senses are senses.

"First comes rhythm," he continues, "because everyone does things in rhythm. People move around to rhythm—like Native American music, Voodoo in Haiti, chain-gang songs, marching bands—and get into a kind of trance. After a while, it becomes so much part of you that it's an invisible thing really.

"Composers use rhythm as background to the other elements. Take Beethoven's *Moonlight Sonata*, the rhythm in the middle movement"—he hums a few bars—"it goes on for about two minutes, puts you in a kind of hypnotic state, then disappears and becomes part of your unconscious. A masterly use of rhythm, where it's not a dominant thing.

"The melody emerges, then harmony and all the other musical elements. If I didn't have those elements, my memory would have nothing to remember. There's a special sensitivity involved—nuances, shading, have to come from the performer playing, it's not in the score."

I ask him what he is especially sensitive to in music, and he replies, "I see colours in music, just as Scriabin did. My mother was an amateur painter, and there were always discussions at home about art and trips to art galleries. When I was a kid, I'd look at a fence and hear a chord: It would actually glow. And I would remember that glow along with the chord."

I'm delighted and confide that my son also hears/sees colours in sound. He replies: "Many people are like that—that's what led me to understand that all the senses are connected. Maybe even before there were human beings, all the senses were one.

"For example, I can understand how someone is feeling because I hear the tension in a person's voice as a kind of coloured texture and can remember the quality of people's voices from years ago—my father and mother, brother and sister, all of them dead now. I *listen*, and then comes the *picture* of the person."

"Will you remember the particular person, too, not just their state of being, even though you might not remember their name?" I ask.

"The person, yes, but I won't remember the name. When I used to recollect names I could hear the sound associated to each name like a kind of music that implanted itself. Now, with deafness, I can still hear the sound, but it doesn't make the same impact. For names to stick, I have to make a strong effort, which I'm not always up to. But I recall a great deal about people—what interests them, what they look like, how they come across, a kind of energy—it's very hard to put into words."

I comment that Callum used to ask, "Must there be words?" about the sensory. "He calls it 'trying to put legs on a snake.' Awareness of someone's energy and remembering the essence of a musical phrase—that seems to be the same sort of thing as the way an artist paints the spaces between the leaves, not the leaves."

"That's a good way of putting it," Meyer agrees, as he pours us another coffee. "Someone said that art is making the invisible visible, bringing in a dimension that is not obvious. Rhythm is obvious, everybody has it. Senses are obvious, automatic. Form, intellect are *not* obvious."

"Okay, Meyer, to come back to our own experience, here we are, both looking at the harbour from your front porch: whose memory of it will be correct? Yours or mine?"

"Memory can't be correct. Facts can be correct, to a certain extent. You can say a drink of water tastes cool, but I don't know what cool means to you, only you know.

"Let's put it this way," he continues. "Whatever way something is conveyed to you—music, art, a person's characteristics—you're only going to remember it if it has some sort of significance for you, a meaning that relates to your life."

"So for you, whatever form music takes—rhythm, melody, colour—you're still going to associate the music to some aspect of your life."

"Well, it's been there from the beginning," he laughs; "it's how I made my living!"

When I ask him what kinds of gigs he's played, Meyer confides that it was pretty tricky earning a living with music, and so he did anything and everything, from symphony appearances to clubs around the state, and much further away. He remembers his first gigs as pianist in the pit for silent movies, which gave him the experience to accompany other performers, such as vocalists and small string ensembles. He made a lot of connections, and eventually his chief source of income was selling musical instruments. True to form, he shrugs off my curiosity about the details of his career—"It isn't very interesting." He is thankful now: he and Miriam had made enough to get by "thriftily, but well enough" in retirement, and, despite his increasing deafness, he can still listen to music and occasionally perform. But what stirs him to the depths of his being is trying to make sense of the world and the way people behave.

Seeing

"It all started at the end of the war: I saw a woman polishing the one window remaining in a bombed-out building in Europe when I was in the U.S. armed forces. I can still hear the squeak of the rag, her eyes staring ahead, not looking at the marching troops or the tanks rolling by.

"Why was she doing that? The building was wrecked; no one could live there. It seemed useless, but she was trying to make some meaning out of her life by doing something familiar. The war was over, she was free. We gave the kids candy, but it made them sick, just like the canned meat we gave the parents. They wanted it, but they couldn't eat it; it was too rich, they'd had nothing like it for years. There we were, the big liberators, feeling good, and they were cheering us. We knew nothing. We thought they would be happy and that would be it. But where were they going to live? Where would they find food? Even cook it? We didn't think of that. It came right down to their daily life and what that meant and how much we didn't know about any of it. We had no understanding, no *sense* of what they'd been through and would go through for years. We were too caught up in being victors. How could we know, coming from a country that hadn't had a war in a hundred years? From then on, all of my life has been a search for meaning, in my own mind, in reading, in listening to other people, in any way I can.

"That woman in the window showed me in a way that no book ever could that human beings are always making meaning, even unconsciously. Like all living beings, we say *yes* to what is nourishing and *no* to what isn't. She was trying to fit into an old meaning-pattern—but it hadn't got through to her that it wasn't going to work."

"Do you think other people in similar situations sometimes try to make sense of them by referring to some external force, such as religious teachings about how suffering makes you a better person and gets you into heaven?" I ask.

"People who say this don't know much about suffering!" he laughs ruefully, "although thinking like that sometimes makes them feel secure. I'm not knocking wanting to feel secure. Who doesn't? It's a chaotic world out there. But the big question is how a person makes a meaningful, liveable existence in a world that could blow up tomorrow. This planet could blow up anytime. That's a fact. *I can't shut that out.* But so many people today are living *all the time* by shutting out. Escaping. I think the greatest gift we have is consciousness, and I feel good whenever I understand something, and grateful. Living or dying, you need to know what's going on in you to be able to cope with the world."

For Meyer, "awareness is like a light. You're in a room, and all the shades are down. You raise a shade and there's the kind of pleasure you feel that goes with wisdom. It demands a kind of control, in that you have to put your emotions on the back burner, so you can *see* something."

When I ask him how he relates his understanding to day-to-day living he answers, a little impatiently, "the relationship is larger than that; there is a kind of brotherhood of seeing. People are like passengers on ships passing one another in the dark and waving to each other in this journey through the fog that is life. I wave to somebody who has overcome fear or cowardice, to someone who is looking for the truth. I appreciate the one who is using his mind. Emotions block seeing and solving problems because they distort things by putting the ego at the centre, as in 'I want something that I'm not getting.' Then we can't see the bigger picture."

"But a lot of what is memorable to you seems to be related to feeling, to people who meant something to you."

"No, I *see* something. I wouldn't call it emotion; it's understanding. It's satisfying. They've meant something qualitatively, even though they may not have been very close emotionally."

What Meyer means by "seeing" confuses me, until I realize that he is using it in several ways. To help me sort this out, I ask him what the difference is for him between qualitative and quantitative. He responds with an example, telling me that he finds people easy to remember because of a quality that emanates from them, but that he isn't good on quantity at all, like remembering a grocery list. For him that's rote memory, which doesn't require any kind of understanding, and he and Miriam write things down or use a mnemonic. "In either case, you're not specifically remembering the things you want to remember but some kind of code, very useful for people studying law or anatomy," he says. "At one stage in my life, I learned how to do it. I used to like to baffle people. That doesn't interest me anymore. It doesn't serve any purpose for me now. It would just be a trick. I'm more interested in how things actually are. What's forgettable is what doesn't relate to that."

Facing Facts

Miriam and I took a break to do the dishes, Meyer grabbed a dishtowel, grinning as he said that most people, including himself, remember what is pleasurable and discard what isn't (like doing the dishes)—but that *life is not like that at all*. He thinks the struggle between liking and disliking is "a disease of the mind" but it's possible to transcend that, "like those gulls looking down and seeing everything that's going on below. Maybe I'm naive, but I think every human being has the potential to transcend the conditions of his life—if only temporarily. I feel that the fate of this world depends on that."

I am finally getting it! His evocative pictorial images—people resemble ship's passengers passing in the dark, the woman in the window, the birds looking down—were making an impact on me (I am more of a visual than an auditory thinker), and I realize that for him "seeing" in the sense of understanding isn't just intellectual, it can be visual, or auditory, can involve all the senses. As if reading my mind, he continues: "To answer your question about separating mind and emotions, it's the great geniuses, to come back to music, who gratify both your feelings *and* your seeing. I have no trouble with feeling. You're feeling all the time, there's no problem there—one's angry, one's frustrated, one's gratified."

"You mean—feelings can be so chaotic, and daily life so endlessly difficult, that a person needs some sort of order to make sense of it all? When I make a sculpture out of a big lump of clay, that's what it feels like I'm doing. It's like Jean Anouilh said, 'Life … lacks form. It's the aim of art to give it some.' You look for the patterns," I add.

"That's it. The woman I saw cleaning the one window left in that bombed-out town, the meaning is not just the window; it's the whole environment and the thoughts that go with it. Here is all of this destroyed, and here is this human being trying to make a little meaning out of this horrible destruction for herself and her people. You have to have seen that destruction for it to have meaning. That's the trouble with meaning. If people don't have the experience, or they don't have the imagination … you're up the wall. You can't create the imagination, you have to *be* imaginative."

"And to have as much experience as possible?" I ask.

"Yes! Either that, or be able to enter empathetically into another person's experience," he replies. "That's what the author, the painter, the musician is after, for you to enter into their experience. Rubenstein, he says he knows he's talking to seven people out of 300. Why should that be?" He looks at me, eyebrows aloft, creasing his forehead.

Asking Questions

"So, what do you think?" I ask.

"I think the education system is partly to blame, because it focuses on teaching to pass tests instead of exposing children to a wide range of experiences, or teaching them about other people so that they can understand and empathize, like asking students to summarize a plot and list characters—that cuts out the meaningful parts. You can use a mnemonic or memorize for tests, then forget it. That's what I did. Anybody can do that. Tests supply information, and that's useful for a lot of things. I want a doctor who knows what he's doing when he sets a broken bone. But where are the questions? You have to have questions."

"Is it questions that keep our minds alive?" I ask, as I watch the dishwater swirling down the sink (and wonder about the septic system).

"Yes, because the questions of life are never fully answered, that's what's so marvellous about them and makes life interesting—and exciting." He reads me a passage from George Seldes' *The Great Thoughts*, about what the great questioners had to say.

"When you read that kind of book, you begin to muse, to wonder, to ask other kinds of questions, don't you?"

"That's right! You make contact with the individual. I'm as close to people who lived 2,000 years ago as if they were alive today. I'll think it over and make additions like 'he didn't know what we know now,' and so on." *(I'd love Meyer to know that I often have inner conversations with him.)*

"Having a conversation with the writer, you're going to remember it because you have half the conversation already."

"That's it! That's how I read. Talking to a person within the context of when he lived."

"But it's important to have a community now, as well as from the past."

"Certainly, you have to interact and make contact now. Passing tests gets you a degree; but there's nothing. No conversation, no understanding, no meaning."

"What you're saying is that it's fundamental to experience as much as possible, on your own, through other people or empathetically, through reading, music and art, to find the patterns that create some kind of order to make sense of our lives and connect us to each other."

"OK. Now [now that I get it, we can go on to the next question!] what is experience?"

Sensory Awareness

Sensory awareness classes were held in the white clapboard one-room schoolhouse standing on the rocks at the south end of the island overlooking the ocean. It is a favourite place for sunset watching, one of the highlights of any visit to the island, and just across the road from Meyer and Miriam's cottage, where we were settling in on the porch to watch it. Classes, the island and the people I met there led to major changes in my life, but when I first met Meyer and Miriam, I was a novice so I asked them what they had learned about sensory awareness in their studies on the island. Meyer was quick to reply, "Well, sensory awareness is basic, only a lot of people don't realize that."

"Basic in the sense that before you can understand anything you must be aware of it in a sensory way?"

"You're a good student," Meyer grins. "In their classes, you begin to see—because they get you to experience it—just how much our organism is very unattended to in this cockeyed world. We're up here in our head, so the energy is there all the time. I wrote a piece, 'Where Is Breathing?' about how to turn our attention to it, like they've been doing in the Orient for thousands of years. When I pay attention to breathing"—he pauses, eyes inward—"it drops where it should be"—takes a full minute. "All this takes time, tranquility; you can't do it and talk. Sitting and quiet, letting go." He sits silently, absorbed in the moment, as I do, wrapped in stillness.

After a while, almost whispering, I ask him, "But how you *communicate* this kind of sensory experience almost has to be non-verbal, through art, music, and the like?"

"Yes. Like Callum said, 'It's like trying to put legs on a snake; the more mind there is, the less sensory communication there will be.'"

We speak of ways to wash away the Zen "monkey mind" of likes and dislikes. Meyer describes how he becomes very quiet so that he can sense. After a while he will observe a change, things look clearer, he hears more sharply, as something comes into awareness. "I had an experience in a class many years ago. We were asked to circle a chair and bow to it. First and second time around I said, 'Why do I have to bow to this damned chair?' The third time, the chair took on a personality of its own. I saw that there was no other chair just like that chair, just like there's no other person like any other, no other leaf, no other … and I bowed to it. And glad to do it. It's the personality of the object that your really rare painter tries to capture."

"So, you must forget about yourself to be able to receive something and in the process find yourself. For you, personality is a constructed thing, a composite of the conditions into which you were born, what you've been taught since childhood. There's an invisible 'true self' unmarked by 'personality.'"

"You got it! We are not born with an *image* of ourselves, only *we* make images of ourselves, not in a personal way—it's a social thing, a made thing. You can't forget it, but it's possible for your image, your ego, to take a back seat once in awhile."

"To be open, to open yourself up like this, Meyer, is to make yourself vulnerable, and that takes a kind of trust."

"Like a child who can trust his mother. But if he hasn't had that kind of trust, he'll be like a swimmer who can't trust the ocean and has to struggle through it. If I had that I wouldn't be concerned with these questions at all, any more than a fish is, who doesn't have to struggle to swim."

Meyer had made it clear from the outset that his private life was off limits, so instead of probing I ask him whether not being able to trust what's happening in our lives makes us question things. He replies, "Either you ask questions or else you just accept every knock, just lie down and let things happen to you."

Old Age and Sensory Memory

We walked over to the schoolhouse to watch the sun go down over the far islands. Meyer settled on a rock big enough to accommodate his gimpy leg and said that what helped him to "struggle his way through life" is not only his questioning mind but also his work on sensory awareness. The aches and pains and daily grind of old age mean he seldom makes a move without discomfort, but when he focuses on his breathing or on the leaves moving in the breeze, he can transcend that. Then he relaxes, understands himself better, and can ignore what the world expects of him, can even sometimes see the parts of himself hiding under "the layers of falsity built up since childhood." He thinks it's essential for people to peel off these layers to discover their senses.

I remembered Alice Miller's account of how she did this in *Pictures of a Childhood* and ask him whether once he begins to peel away those layers he'll remember something meaningful from the past.

Like most people, he remembers significant things. But *why* they were significant is a matter of "excavating the unconscious.

"I'll give you another example from the war that I've reflected on over the years. We were liberating a concentration camp in Bavaria and then putting people who broke curfew in prison. I felt this was wrong and went to the officer. He didn't understand that at all, he had no *sense* of how these people were feeling, couldn't make any contact at all, at any level, not even in his mind. All he knew were orders. That's bureaucracy: the individual is buried, becomes a machine—orders—another test he memorized, couldn't hear a question, couldn't ask one."

"That's something you'll never forget."

"No."

As we watch sky and water meet in blazing red I ask him how *he* reflects on things, peels away the layers, until he is aware of another level of experience and memory. He answers, "I lie in bed in that state between sleeping and waking and let my thoughts wander: It's like a question's been asked that concerns me during the night, something about what I saw or how I behaved. And I'll see some answer to it; it'll all come out clearly."

As with Emma in her story "Coming Home," his unconscious is working on it during the night.

"I'll know there's something unsatisfying about it, something that doesn't feel right, and then be aware of other things surrounding it, which I don't have to go into now. You just see something and you think, 'Oh yeah, that's good.' I lie there for a while thinking that over, and then I feel a certain clarity."

"You know, Meyer, for a while I was confused about what you mean by 'seeing.' You use that word in several different contexts, and at first I thought you meant understanding intellectually. It wasn't until I got on to how pictorial you are, that I began to understand."

Meyer looks puzzled, not understanding what I mean by pictorial, and I explain that he paints verbal pictures to illustrate what he means.

He looks even more baffled. "Pictures? What pictures?" he asks.

"Well, let's see. You started out with the woman in the window. I'm not going to forget that either, or the concentration camp. Then there's awareness being like a light in a dark room, and people who understand each other like passengers waving on a ship, and transcending ego like a bird looking down, and then trust being like a fish who doesn't have to struggle to swim. There are probably more."

"It's just a way of speaking," he shrugs, but I point out that it's such a good example of how all the senses are related that it has me wondering whether he makes an emotional attachment to the visual as well as the auditory. "I remember that you said that sounds have colour for you and how an 'experience moves something in you.' I mean, what I understand now is that no matter what you see—it could be understanding the shape of things, a pattern, or a non-verbal sensory message communicated in meditation, or through one of the arts, or an insight filtering up through the unconscious or in a relationship, the payoff …"

"… is always the clarity."

"Like a picture," I add.

"OK, OK. I get your point. You have a way of persisting, don't you?"

"It takes one to know one!"

"Oh, does it!" he laughs. "I guess it does ..."

A Long Life
Old Age and the Gift of Life

"... Well, anyway, you see, I can say, no matter how old I am, or what my physical condition might be, in all likelihood I'll have that clarity until the last moment—unless I'm on drugs. I'm willing to accept the fact that when consciousness stops that's the end. Until that moment I feel gratitude. We began with an accident, in a simple one-celled creature a billion years ago, under certain climatic conditions. Nobody knows why it happened there, and not someplace else. And you don't have to know. In my book, the greatest sin is ingratitude for the gift of life. To me, that's unbearable. Watching people walk around just focusing on themselves, not realizing how fortunate they are to live in this country: taking everything for granted is like a smell in the air that I can't push away." He deals with it by focusing on what is "real and living, that's why people are important to me. Reading or talking with them brings out all kinds of stuff in me that I might not think of by myself; I get more clarity. The pleasures of the mind, to meet a fine mind, it all increases my understanding of what life is about. This feeds back to what I said before: only human beings make meaning."

"And they make it together!"

"Definitely."

I remembered how he talked to people on the road every day, and then of how important people are to Martha in "working through" her feelings about the hurts of her childhood, her growing up, and her marriage and ask Meyer if peeling away the layers and finding out what matters improves with practice as one ages.

"It becomes irrelevant. You go through life, and you find that 99 out of 100 times your grudges, rejections from childhood, your career, your marriage are a mistake, or wanting to impress someone, or your own misconceptions."

Thinking of Russell and of how his bitterness about lost opportunities undercut his achievements and his pleasure in them, I ask Meyer about the two-edged sword of memory: treasuring one's experiences, learning from them as one remembers, yet the hurt that can come, especially if disappointments and losses pervade one's life.

"If you take the step of dropping it—and that's not just one step, it's an ongoing thing—you find that the world is not out there to do you in. The world is a lot better place, people are a lot better than the institutions and the politicians and the bureaucrats who take advantage of them."

"But you still have to dig down into your unconscious, as you say, to be able to do that."

"Oh, yes. You do. And not everyone wants to do that," he laughs.

Lessons on Being Old

We walk back to the cottage as the indigo afterglow deepens at day's end. As we watch our steps carefully on the dirt road Meyer says, "You see, our youth-oriented culture needs lessons on being old. There are books and courses on every stage of human development, lots of information about financial planning, housing, and health care for people in their 50s, and books about how adult children can care for older people without burning out.

"All of this is important," he comments, "but where are the books and courses about *being* old? People need information on how to deal with superficiality, what the culture tells you is important but isn't any longer—if it ever was, and on staving off the boredom of daily tasks by focusing on the value of the people and events themselves. I would like to have known more about how to compensate for deafness and back and leg problems, like this"—lifting his cane—"*before* they happened. When you're already in pain, it's hard to learn how to get beyond it so you can appreciate your past, and what you have now, and enjoy what you can't have vicariously without turning sour."

"That's a pretty tall order! How do you handle the daily drag?"

"*Being old is a tall order*" he fires back. "I'm still learning how to deal with it. The first thing is to get beyond the habit of gossip so you can ask questions. If you take the time to listen to people they'll think you're a great conversationalist, even if you haven't said a word except to ask a question now and again. And you might learn something. A lot of people are more interesting than they seem at first. Finding something that is significant *right now*, you need all the help you can get. That's why old people tend to remember the past more. It *means* more. Your thoughts can wander in the present because you've heard it many times before."

"You mentioned questioning as a way to keep life interesting, and Miriam talks about ways to make things fresh."

"We work on it; we keep on reminding ourselves that no sensation is ever the same, that walking down the road today is not the same as yesterday. If you don't, you'll find yourself saying, 'What the hell, I've done that so many times.' And then you'll start to forget. Especially if it's harder to do— which it usually is. Maybe you used to prance down the road. Or maybe there are a lot of unpleasant memories connected to it, like you pass a house and someone's not there who used to be there, and you'd like them to be there. The older you get, the more these subtle things come up from down below."

"Our senses get duller as we age so you need to train the other senses to be more acute," I comment.

"Yes, and instead of condemning myself when I have distracting thoughts, I ask myself to become aware of the distraction and focus on the present. You look out the window, see the movement of branches. I may be getting more freshness now, more seeing now, than when I was four years old. It's a willful thing. I tell myself, 'I don't want to walk through this world in a semi-daze, waiting until the end,' like so many old people. I also try to remember the things I used to do with a kind of empathy, and, like I said, enjoy those memories by entering into them imaginatively."

We pause to light the coal-oil lamps and sink in to the easy chairs by the fire—it gets cold quickly on the island at night. Picking up the conversation I ask, "Do older people have an advantage in this kind of 'vicarious enjoyment'?"

"Sure, we can draw on our own experience to identify with another person—a ballet dancer, or even a bird or a tree. You may not be able to do much more, but you *can* appreciate it."

"That's what a good writer does, Meyer, don't you think?" I add. "And an attentive reader too. After all, how can you read great literature if you can't do that? It grows, doesn't it? Like Martha says, when one thing is clarified something else surfaces."

"Yes, it does. She's a quiet one. I don't agree with her about religion, but we've had some interesting conversations. You also learn from experiencing that certain things you've done, or have a tendency to do, have consequences, are maybe destructive. You don't want that. I'm talking about me now; some people don't seem to want to give up their negative attitudes. This is a personal matter. Ten, 20 years ago I might not have wanted to talk about this with you. In fact, my first feeling was *not* to, because I have a built-in antagonism for surveys and questionnaires that don't go anywhere."

"And you prefer to go towards something? If you can?"

"You have a conflict here. Talking about this sort of thing takes energy and will power, because sometimes you're not up to par. Very often it's just easier to get away from the whole life situation, especially when you're old and you know the end is coming. You can say, 'Well, I'll just pull the blanket over my head and wait 'til the end,' or 'I'll just sit here and let these nice nurses do their thing,' and you're not really awake or alive. Or you can open your eyes and see something. When you see something, there are changes."

"It seems to me, Meyer, that being open to your experiences is what life is about, no matter how old you are."

"Yes, but make no mistake: *being old makes a difference.* There's something in us that prepares us for the end. You *know.* You know it from one year to the next. You know you have less energy, and that you have to accept it, or use up more energy railing about having had a miserable life."

Remembering Florida Scott-Maxwell again—that her heart must be a miracle of quiet to endure the intensity of her life—I ask Meyer how he handles the intensity of his everyday experiences with diminished energy.

"It depends on the experience," he says. "While you can't have the experiences of a young person, you can remember similar experiences and at least talk their language, make those contacts that are so important as you age. Otherwise you'd have nobody to talk to!" he quips, adding (as Lev, Miriam, and Martha do), that "there's an emotional drive I don't need any more, I'm quieter now. I don't need to—don't want to, really—live that way anymore. I can be satisfied now to just identify to some extent with other people or with the wind blowing through those leaves and branches. It's only if you turn your attention to it that you get better at it, no matter what your age. I'm not kidding myself; if I have a political discussion with someone I'm not being aware, I'm making points. That's my choice, either I want to be quiet or I want to be verbal and have the gratification of winning points and satisfying my ego. It's just that now I'm more aware that that's what I'm doing."

"It sounds like you understand yourself differently now."

He looks at me wistfully, "Yes, from my earliest days on, I was influenced by the great thinkers whose works I read. I remember thinking then that wherever they went I was willing to go. But it was a lonely place for a young man. Now I realize that they too had spent their whole lifetimes thinking about the same issues as I do; I feel a sense of comradeship, that I'm part of 'the brotherhood of seeing' and don't feel so isolated."

Giving the Ego a Back Seat

It's getting late and time to leave. Miriam sets out cookies to go with our evening tea as I tease, "Do we have sisters in this gang too?" Meyer's eyebrows lift, "Of course! It's just a way of speaking. If I don't make the effort to understand myself, I'd be batting my head against the wall—it takes a long time. Besides, there's so much going on in the world that change is going to come very slowly, maybe not in our lifetime. But, the older I get, the more I experience a sense of wonder.

"Scientific exploration amazes me, everything from the brain to outer space, knowledge of the very small and enormously big—I don't want to exclude any of the wonders—I just have to try to be fearless and say, 'Well, OK, I am grateful for my awareness of this. I don't know what it means, I may never know.'

"Even though I'm deteriorating physically, I want *to break through this closing in* that can come with age. I don't feel any older in my mind or my spirit; I live from day to day with whatever enjoyment is there. And when one has a sense of wonder, death is not at all a fearful thing. If I didn't wake up tomorrow, that would be OK, as far as I'm concerned: it's the end of consciousness, that's all."

Facing Old Age and Death

"'*This closing in*.' That's a wonderfully expressive way of visualizing old age, Meyer. What does it take to face this fearlessly, in a universe where the individual is not very important?"

"Well, there are two ways. First, it's important to know that your ego is a put-together thing, that you're not born with it, and that something that is put together can be taken apart. All the great ones have said that."

"That's a tough proposition."

"I don't think you're going to find many converts to this at all"—we are both laughing.

"It's much easier to share your complaints and grievances with someone," Meyer says. "'Misery loves company': there's a lot of truth in that. Or spend your time wanting to be important. You do that, there's no room for appreciating the wonders of the universe—including the wonder that is consciousness. I like to think that everyone has the potential, that when you can work through the obstacles, you can reach this sense of wonder. But that's very hard for some older people when the realities of their lives become insurmountable."

"Is knowing you can change your perspective one of the good things about being old?"

"Anyone who is poor, or sick, or lonely and old is not in a good position—let's be practical about that. Those are your preoccupations. They have to be. I consider us very fortunate, Miriam and me. We know this. With a little help she can function at home, we can afford that. There's nothing good in itself about being old, or about being young, for that matter. You don't see the youth going around just blooming with joy. They're full of problems. There's nothing good or bad about any age. You have to make your way in a very complex world that is not at all interested in you growing or realizing yourself. A truly civilized society would be concerned with every individual realizing himself, but so far we don't have that."

"Do you think a middle-aged person like me can really grasp what's coming next?"

"Well, you need to understand about loss. Loss is a big one. Growing old, you lose pieces of yourself you always took for granted. Your hearing goes, your eyesight, your mobility, and you have to adjust to that. I'm bringing it up again because it's hard for a younger person to grasp how important this is— and you may not think so, but you're still young. Then there's, well, people who meant something to you, or move away to be closer to family. We have nieces and nephews. We spent a lot of time with them when they were younger. Now, of course, they're grown, with families of their own. And some of them have older parents to look after too. But we're all right; we can still do things together, although we can't get out as much, especially at night.

"Miriam tires easily since her stroke. She used to enjoy going to the store and the post office to shop and hear the news. That would be her day's outing now. I used to walk to the cliffs, or the woods. Not now. The effort to climb to the bluffs, especially coming downhill with a foot and leg brace, makes it almost impossible. But my feet remember every twist and bend on the trail, and I can hear the surf breaking on the cliffs, feel that exhilaration."

"Is there a big difference between 70 and 80?"

"Yes, even between 75 and 80 I tired more and more quickly, and my treasured hearing seems to worsen. For a musician like me, that's the worse loss."

"I hate to think there will be no more singsongs with Dora and the gang."

"We'll do it as long as we can. You know, these impairments diminish your sense of accomplishment; that's very hard, that one! As I said, it's hard for the need for security and a sense of wonder to coexist!"

"You spoke of two things that stand in the way of a sense of wonder, your ego and—what's the other one?"

"There's something that has to be said here. We talked about the marvels of memory, and that's true. Without memory, there is no consciousness and no way to have any meaning in your life, let alone make a living, or even get along from day to day. On another level, you're not going to be free of your ego—that stands between you and a sense of wonder—unless you are free of the baggage of memory."

"What kind of baggage?"

"The stuff you hang on to. We talked about that last week, all those hurts and resentments, memories of what could have been and now never will be. You know, that promotion you thought you should have had, an old flame, things about your family—which you couldn't have changed anyway."

"Miriam says there are things you never forget but that you must 'file and forget,' put them out of your mind," I observe.

"You're right; that stuff can take up a lot of space."

"Are there attachments and associations involved with memory that get in your way of 'seeing' things?"

"Absolutely," he sighs. "A young child has not made those attachments yet, is innocent. Old age is not like infancy, that loss of memory is something different. Looking out of innocent eyes when you're old can mean that person has Alzheimer's, for all you know."

"So you're saying that to experience wonder an older person has to subtract a lot. You might say forget. If she can. Then she might be able to re-experience that sense of wonder?"

"Subtract a lot for sure, yeah, but it's not the same. Because it involves a kind of appreciation a younger person can't have, they haven't experienced enough yet. And that's a big 'if' you're talking about. The psychological grooves that our culture sets up are not so easily disposed of. You have to put something in its place if you're going to be free of that memory, then you can thank whatever you want to thank for what you have, and use it as much as you can, and be aware of what's going on in you that stands in the way. That's a whole course in itself."

"I think you could teach that course, Meyer! What is the most important aspect of memory for you?"

"To me the importance of memory is what you can learn from it—yours or somebody else's. Trial and error. Doing that caused this, so I'm not going to do that. You are either learning or you're dying."

"You're alive!"

"You're alive, you have consciousness. At the last moment, you can still have some of your senses. Even if it's only a memory of some of them, you can still see the contours of existence, the colours, the shapes. And you relate to them all. So, to me, memory is looking over all of that, from the very earliest age, knowing you did the best you could under the circumstances. You know that a feeling of hostility in you is destructive. That's what memory is to me. At least, that's what I'm thinking right now. A record of the past and learning something. It doesn't matter how old you are, are you learning something? And it's important to say that we are not alone in this world, what others do and say interacts with our experience. That's why you must keep on asking what is true for you, not as a theory, but for you as a person. I don't think it's the same for everybody. What is true is the sense of what makes me alive. Asking, 'When am I alive?'"

"When are we alive, Meyer?"

"When we're breathing!"

"Oh, Meyer, that's what you said earlier, didn't you? Senses are senses! You know, Miriam said something like that a while ago about how a sense of well-being is basic to all the rest."

"That too, that too."

Awareness: A poem for Meyer

We are passengers on ocean-going ships
travelling through the dark, waving
to each other in a flash of recognition
mouths ready to speak,

sometimes like high-flying birds
we penetrate the fog
of daily struggle, prisoners to a silly ego
bound to passing whims, and see

a window standing alone in a worn-out wall,
polished to a sheen by hope.
Microscopic
or the big picture, we gaze in wonder ...

... a fence glows blue in a D minor chord,
shines red to high C
sounds as brilliant as the morning light when
the shutters open

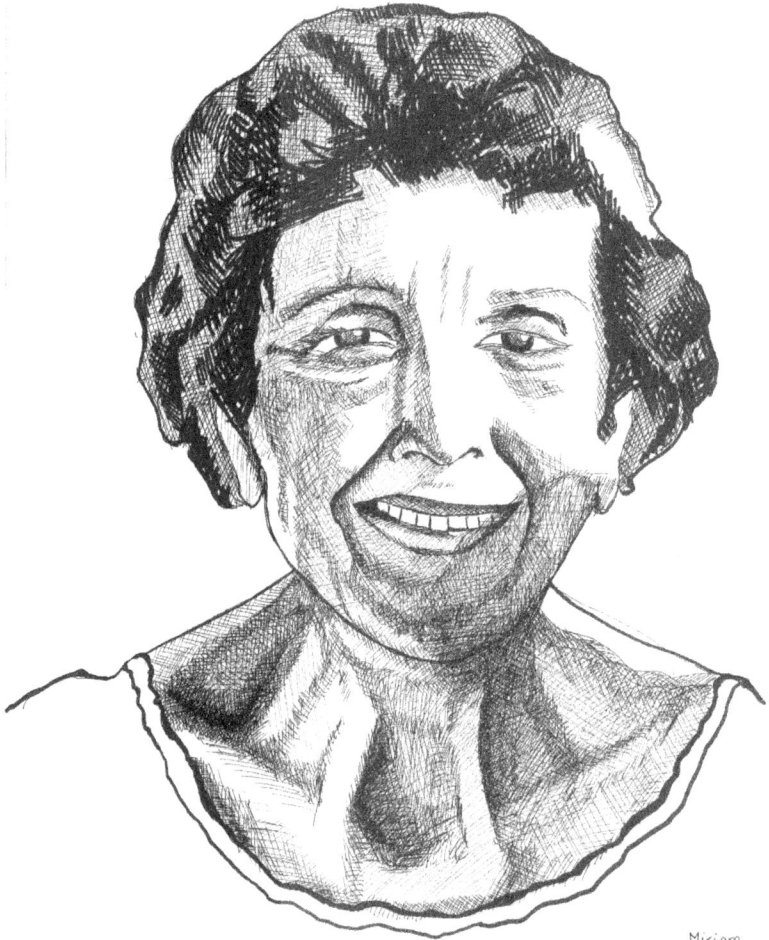

Miriam

The Nuts and Bolts of Everyday Life: Miriam's Story

"We are made up of the times we are born into."

She lay on the floor all night, a blanket covering her, a pillow under her head; she remembers Meyer's alarmed face bending over her and trying to speak to him with her eyes. At six in the morning, just as soon as he knew someone would be up, Meyer walked over to the bed and breakfast where one of the island's emergency response squad lived; the crew came with a stretcher and carried Miriam down to the fishing boat on standby. By the time they got to shore, and then on an ambulance to the nearest hospital, the stroke was well advanced. There was not much for her to do except learn— slowly and laboriously, and with all the determination her broken body and weakened will could muster—how to deal with the damage. And learn she did.

For the first time in more than 50 years of marriage she was deeply angry with Meyer that endless night. In all their years together his dependence on her had irritated her plenty of times, more exasperation really. But that night, when she was so helpless that he couldn't ask her what to do, her exasperation changed to anger, and then fear. She tried. Tried to show him her fear and urgency with her eyes. One time she was able to move her hand towards the door—it's still her good hand—but he didn't see. He looked so worried, stroked her head trying to comfort her, but he didn't understand. She remembers feeling hopeless, the sinking feeling, even as she was drifting in and out of consciousness, because she'd have to wait—no chance of getting the drug they can give you in the first few hours.

"Meyer thinks he's sensitive to people's emotions. He isn't. He's sensitive to how they use their minds. He's always relied on me to remind him people have emotions. He can talk when you get emotions out of the way."

"He can certainly get pretty heated when he's trying to persuade someone," I say; "can sound almost hectoring." Miriam laughs, saying he doesn't realize that even at his most passionate he thinks he's being reasonable and other people aren't. "You see, I was brought up to notice things, to watch people. Observation is something I do, have always done. It's not thought, which is about ideas, it's about the nuts and bolts of everyday life."

Learning to Understand People

I first met Miriam on a Thursday morning, the day the catch arrived fresh at the Fish House, a small grey shack tucked in a sheltered corner on the harbour shore. A short, attractive, grey-haired woman with a round face and gentle smile, we would chat a little, and then eventually, at my request, she showed me how to choose the best fish. I've been cooking scallops her way ever since she showed me how, that suppertime by coal-oil lamp.

When we get to know each other better she tells me a little about her background. She was brought up by her older sister Ria while her mother worked. She looked up to Ria as a model, even though she was "emotionally unreliable"—Miriam never knew when or how she would do something her sister thought was wrong and would punish her by not sewing her clothes or by not talking to her. She learned how to "mind her Ps and Qs," watching every move, listening to every word, learning empathy through "being attentive to the person," knowing that only watching and tightly controlling her emotions kept her from being manipulated by her sister, and her mother.

Self-directed from the beginning, she grew up feeling alone. Even now, she can't always trust her emotions because they'll "well up and get in the way of understanding." And she has always had a hard time trusting other people's emotions because she's found they, like her sister's resentment, can be capricious and hurtful. To this day she wants to "shut overly emotional people out of my life, past and present. Remembering them is terrible, like looking through dark glasses all the time."

One of those dark times: after her stroke people seemed to feel sorrier for Meyer than for her. No one ever asked how *she* felt, lying on the floor all night waiting for him to ask for help. Trying to understand their reaction after her anger died down, she wondered whether people were embarrassed, or guilty about resenting their own mothers being sick or old, when they could see she wasn't strong like they were used to. "It's almost like they felt I had let Meyer down in some way," she said. That's why Miriam doesn't "boast her age" anymore—it seems to put younger people off now; they don't seem glad to see an intelligent 83-year-old, active and strong, even after a stroke. Young people seem to speak a different language and don't want to hear what the old have to say—especially about how you have to take care of yourself as you get older, as she does: "I was intelligent about that even before my stroke, although I maybe took more for granted than I should, counted on my good genes a bit too much."

She remembers the strain of being young, remembers that what she wanted in an older person was a mother, and is pretty sure that the young are attracted to her because that's what they see in her, "especially the men, who want intelligence and strength—but with a certain motherly softness." She doesn't give advice; at least she tries not to. "It doesn't help any. I've lived long enough to know what I know: the language of the old faces reality, sees how people are unwitting victims of social and cultural conditions, made up of the times we are born into."

She tells me that Meyer was attracted to *her* because she had a brain, and that he has always counted on her to listen to his ideas. Now that they've retired she is often his audience, at least in the city where they're alone more; many of their friends have died or, like them, find it harder to get out. They depend on each other for companionship, especially around their shared love of music and books. Every night they read aloud to each other or more often, now that she hasn't as much energy (or fluency) for reading aloud, listen to a book tape and then discuss it. The tapes are clear enough that Meyer can hear the voices, despite his deafness, although they both think that a lot of contemporary writing is "drivel, young people talking about themselves as if they were important."

On the island, where they spend the summer, Miriam gets time by herself when Meyer sets off on errands after breakfast. He's gone for hours, talking to anyone who will listen. "And they do; he's interesting." Miriam says, "I get a lot from him, I have always admired his mind, the way he bores into things, questions, synthesizes and doesn't just consume knowledge."

Homemaker

Even when she was a full-time teacher she provided the setting for weekly get-togethers of friends who enjoyed the intellectual stimulation, as well as the good food she always provided. At island gatherings I've watched her cool Meyer down and lighten the atmosphere, as she puts it, when he is too insistent. She tells me that homemaking is something she's always done and still does. What her friend Callum, another islander, calls "the vital elements of existence," and "having a memory for simple systems" (which he regrets he doesn't have) Miriam has always thought of as coming to her automatically. She watched all the ways her mother made a home and was brought up to expect that she should know these skills and so she doesn't really know how she remembers them—"I just do it."

Miriam's Austrian Jewish parents emigrated during the Depression. Her father was a scholar, the kind of man, as she said, who was married off to a woman who did all the work and supported him. Her parents were lost in America, where there wasn't the same kind of intellectual tradition—that is, that men had the ideas and women worked at a paid job, as well as taking care of all the family's physical needs, raising the children, and making a home. She watched her mother being a drudge her whole life and thought she was dumb to do it. Now she realizes that without education her mother's ignorance left her vulnerable to not knowing any other way than manipulating others, "like playing favourites to get what she wanted because she couldn't get it for herself."

Since homemaking has always come naturally to Miriam she's never thought of it as particularly important or, until lately, as having much to do with memory. What *is* important to her, what she is "glad of" and has come to appreciate so much more as she ages, is her organizational skills, developed and perfected over years of juggling the demands of home and profession. In retirement her expertise helps compensate for gradually diminishing energy so that she can still keep up a good home, "not just cleaning and laundry, but good food and a place where friends can enjoy themselves." Now, with the stroke, she can't cook up a storm anymore: they have people to lunch instead of dinner, she has shortcuts like buying desserts, and Meyer helps out more. While the demands are much heavier on both of them now, he still has more time to "read and reflect" than she does. However, the fact that she is able to do it, that even young people like to visit them, are interested in what they do, brings her a quiet satisfaction and a sense that her life is almost normal. The stroke has restricted her, but since she had already experienced some of the limitations of growing older, the stroke was a shock to her, but not a complete surprise.

Teacher

These are the everyday small triumphs. But looking back over her 83 years Miriam is proudest of her educational achievements as a young woman and of her long career teaching in New York's public school system. She tells me that her "mother got us our education. Our father objected—we'd just marry and raise children—but she knew that education gives you the knowledge and ideas you need to qualify for a profession and make a good living so we wouldn't live a life of drudgery the way she did. And my education and my profession made me into a feminist because men don't keep me, or keep me down. I've always worked. The other [homemaking] is just training, being in touch with people's needs, and that's observation."

"It's work, though, homemaking," I said.

"Yeah, full-time, though it's drudgery, a trap."

"Boring—but you're glad you are good at it."

"Oh sure, it's useful."

"It's taught you a lot though: about organizing your life, about people, given you one of the ways to have a social life?"

"It has, but you know, there, I give to them. To give a lot is my way of winning. Teaching gave me that understanding." She smiles as she recalls her teaching days: teaching by rote, she says, requires more skill than intelligence, and what you learn that way, if you don't use it afterwards, you'll forget the day after the exam. She wanted her students to be excited about the material and knows that her well-honed powers of observation allowed her to become aware of each child and to "understand what their needs were and how they could mesh with the curriculum." As she grew in experience and competence, so did her self-confidence and her assertiveness. The brightest students were the most intriguing: "Teaching them was really teaching," she said, "because I was giving them the ideas and knowledge they needed to get somewhere in life." And they challenged her own knowledge, which kept her on her toes, gave her the intellectual stimulation she's always loved. Watching, listening, guiding, selecting, encouraging—teaching tools and the memory thread of her life.

Miriam left teaching to marry and have a child, but the baby died. The rules at the New York School Board barring married women from teaching had recently been lifted for childless women, but the board was reluctant to rehire her. Being outspokenly assertive has never been her way, and so it wasn't easy for Miriam to insist that they take her back. But she did insist, and they had to relent or break the rules. Then, when she was given a class no one wanted, of "lower-class kids who weren't too bright," she knew they were trying to push her out. "That's how they punished you." *(For losing the baby? For daring to come back? For not living up to a [middle-class] ideal of fertile womanliness? Who was she letting down then?)*

Even though, as immigrants, her family were poor, they came from a middle-class background, and Miriam had always assumed that is where bright kids come from (rightly, in terms of intellectual background and the skills needed to pass exams, as current research shows). She'd always taught that kind of class, so this was new for her. "I had compassion for those kids. I knew how they felt different—my parents did, and I did, as the child of immigrants. But even though we were poor and often went hungry we had the example of my father, always studying, talking to us at dinner—he had to; there were no boys." She knows she did a good job of teaching her students. She got the parents—which really meant the whole community—involved in their children's education so they'd know what was going on and could help them. But she wouldn't have chosen that class because she enjoyed the bright ones so much. "I know I ought not to be critical, but it's hard for me to tolerate people who aren't bright and alert."

Keeping Her Mind Fresh

After retirement, Miriam continues to takes courses to "keep her mind fresh," as she says, and is pleased to find that she can still pass an exam with the best of them, and take part in any discussion. She has a low opinion of the adult educators who can't be bothered to understand their students. She's often encountered that kind of teacher, for whom adult education is just "an add-on job," and so they don't really care about the students. I comment that she's had a very different attitude, and she replies that she realizes that her lower-class children taught her how to be a real teacher, focusing on how to interest students in ideas, no matter their background or origins.

Miriam thinks that remembering ideas and accumulating knowledge are intentional: you have to want to remember, and motivating children to want to know something is what teaching is all about. She thinks that intentional memory is recalling what you were conscious of, what you paid attention to; "it's not something that comes with old age at all, but if you've practised it, expect it, or have regard for it." The older she gets the more important it is for her to know what is in "the back of consciousness"—why this particular thought or feeling, and not another. When I ask her if she thought this practice of tuning in to her consciousness was a part of her growth and development, as well as part of the way she lived day-to-day, she replied that you have to orient yourself that way, and that she's made it a purpose in her life since middle age because it influences her personality, her self-awareness, and occasionally her image of herself. "And it can be gratifying."

In Miriam's opinion you pay close attention to what you use, or to what interests you enough to go to the trouble of remembering it, which includes attending to your inner life. She thinks that what you observe through reading, or listening to music, or looking at art is more abstract because it's what other people have observed (although her own responses are often both intuitive and physical). After she's read something, or looked at a painting, or listened to music, she doesn't know if it's going to stay in her mind until she has occasion to tell somebody about it. That's why good conversation is so important to her; it's an occasion for use, and she's more likely now to remember something only when she uses it.

"I don't try to remember, don't consciously store it in my head. If I need to remember something, I do. If I'm not remembering, and I want to, I slow down, become quiet so I can concentrate—it'll come to me. I just let it rest in the back of my head and it will come spontaneously." This is not forgetting, because if someone gives her a hint, she'll remember. As with Lev's key phrase, Avram's image, and Emma's melody, "a word recalls a topic area, and then I'm off!"

While she tells me that she doesn't think about memory very much, or worry about it, just recently she's having regrets about what she calls training herself to forget names when she was young. She remembers modelling herself on an older girl at school who thought it was cute to forget people's names. Now, she doesn't think it's cute anymore, and agrees with Lev that people like it when you remember their names. She's finding it hard to break the habit, so she uses strategies like getting people to introduce themselves to each other or focusing just on the first name. And she can almost always remember something about them, like their job, their family, mutual interests they've talked about, and that will often recall the name.

Miriam thinks that while associating memory loss and aging may sometimes be a fact of life, it's mostly a cliché. She doesn't really care enough about it to look into all the stereotypes and their reasons. She takes a much more practical approach, is more interested in understanding what is happening with her own memory as her life changes. Until very recently she has always thought that the continuous memory thread provided by the structure of the week's routine, and the organizational skills she counts on to remember what she's "always done and still does" is a different, less important, and certainly less interesting kind of memory than the memory of ideas and knowledge provided through advanced education. As she becomes older she realizes just how important that "memory for simple systems" is, because she'll forget things when she hasn't enough energy to be as well organized as she used to be. Boredom can be a factor as well. Like Meyer, Alice and several of the others I talked to, Miriam says that when you age, a lot of what is going on the world *is* boring; you've been there so many times that sometimes people just "let go on life, and so they don't pay attention."

Now much of Miriam's energy and willpower go into another kind of knowledge, learning the skills to recover from her stroke. She knows it's reasonable to expect that she can't do everything she used to do, or have as much energy for outside interests like taking courses, or possess the stamina to be with people so that she has a chance to exercise her mind in a good discussion. But it still exasperates her, because when she's not using her mind she begins to doubt her intelligence, and hence herself. I ask her what she means, and she says she doesn't know whether she could be patient with herself if she thought she was intellectually impaired. I comment that she'd managed to do that with her students, and she laughs a little, saying she's glad she hasn't had to test her tolerance of her own failings in that way, "because it's all there. I can sense it. I'm still bright. It's a matter of calling on other parts of my mind."

I wonder what other parts of her mind she means, and she replies that it's the ones she hasn't used so much, or has taken for granted. Now she needs to discover other ways to express them, and she finds that means using a different kind of brain power. At the very beginning her stroke affected her memory, but that didn't last long after she realized, with great relief, that there was nothing wrong with her intellect. It was just that she was tired a lot, and concentrating really hard to relearn muscular patterns, and to use other senses, took most of her energy and time.

"That's another kind of remembering, isn't it?" I observed—"teaching your muscles to remember how to work. Is that what you mean when you talk about another kind of brain power, about using different parts of your mind?"

"I guess so. That kind of attention, tuning in to your body—it takes a lot of patience."

"Patience, energy—and time!" I respond.

"It sure does. I'm glad I grew up with that. I wasn't glad then, because I had to, but I am now."

"That you learned how to observe, be empathetic—how to tune in to other people? Now it's your turn, to tune in to yourself, I mean."

"That's right. Otherwise you know, I recall everything; I remember the good and the bad. I remember some things too well, and wish I didn't: hurt feelings, being slighted or humiliated by my sister, or knowing what they were saying about the kids, and about me, when they gave me that class, and I don't want to recall it all the time." She tries to forget past hurts by finding reasons, or putting them in perspective, or thinking of what the situation opened up for her. "I try not to dwell on it, not to give it any attention. I put the memory aside, what I call 'file and forget.' That's what you have to do or you'd end up being sad or angry all the time."

"Do you ever forget the anger, though?" I ask.

"Oh no."

"So, what do you do?"

"Well, you learn to recognize it sooner, and to put it in better perspective. And you learn to not let it bother you as much."

"Is that it?" I said in my much younger naiveté.

She looks at me quizzically, smiling a little, and says patiently, but very firmly, "That's enough!"

Down through the years I've given Miriam's words to many people, like the gift they have been to me as I have come to understand that not only is recognizing your emotions, putting them in perspective, and accepting your strengths and limitations enough, but also how hard even this is.

Avoid the Past

For Miriam to learn how to do this, she tells me, she's had to discourage the kind of memory involved in reminiscence, in herself or others. When she talks about tuning in to herself she means the sensations and feelings she is experiencing now. She thinks that classes that have people "dredging up the past" are a bad idea because nostalgia is sentimental, has people remembering the past with regret: "What's the point of that?" she asks. Her early years hold few joys for Miriam. She thinks that to keep on remembering old hurts and grudges, which she could remember only too well if she let herself, is obsessive, unhealthy, not useful, and just upsetting.

She is also greatly disturbed by the current world situation and the terrible wars she says are in no one's interest except power-hungry dictators and greedy multinationals, like arms manufacturers, some of the worst of them in the United States. "I love my country, but I don't know what we're coming to. It scares me; Meyer too. He thinks it's important to remember the past, as in past wars, as a way of being sure to remember certain images that people are only too willing to forget because they don't want to understand why people do these things. It's important to him to try to figure it out, to find the meaning. I don't want to do that."

She knows she will always remember unhappy experiences but she doesn't do it "on purpose," is not what she calls a "compulsive rememberer," like Meyer. She doesn't want to struggle with meaning anymore; she doesn't have the energy, and, besides, there's nothing more she can do—she's not working, not teaching. She wonders how her memories of war and being poor are going to help anyone when no one is interested in hearing them anyway. "No one listens. So, instead of feeling angry or depressed, I try to put it on the back burner and let it go."

She has learned ways to do that, learned that when you get old and you're not working, or you can't get out as much to go to lectures or theatre or to meet people, that it's important to have something new and interesting in your life or your mind. Since retiring she enjoys the more relaxed routine of looking after Meyer and her home, but daily life without the stimulation of work can get boring,

"The days lose their character. I used to hate Sundays."

"Because the next day was the beginning of the week's work?"

"Oh no! Because there was nothing much to do! Unless we were going to a concert, or something like that. Sunday is family day for a lot of people, and we didn't have a family."

So she is always looking for something that lights a spark. Now, with her diminished vitality, she has to juggle that need with fatigue, and with the time and energy it takes to listen to "all the babble I've heard so many times, or wade through all the junk you read, to find something good.

"Like when I met you I thought getting to know a new person might be too much. I already had many friends, but when I heard that you were researching memory and aging I got interested. It wasn't something I'd ever given much thought to before. And then I got to like you because you were lively and interested in everything, like Meyer, wanting to get to the bottom of things. I don't necessarily want to do that myself, but it's intriguing."

"So, let me get this straight," I said. "It's almost impossible for you to forget about what's going on in the world, but current events are so unsettling that you don't want to think about them very much. You find that people can be boring, books trite and repetitious. And you tell me that even the music that you and Meyer have always enjoyed isn't as sustaining as it used to be. So where do you find the freshness that you say you need to stay alert, to nourish you?"

"Nature is never boring, nature never lets me down. Nature is always interesting because there's always something new, if you're open to it and know how to look." Miriam tells me that becoming old, accelerated by the consequences of her stroke, has taught her that the sensory world of nature and her awareness of her sensations and feelings—good and bad, tolerable and intolerable, pleasurable or not—have always been the ground of all memory for her. She has come to see the senses not only as the cumulative source of her memories, but also as a part of the process of memory, of *the way* that she remembers and forgets. While her lifelong interest has been to keep her mind active and her ideas alive and fresh, Miriam has "always known that *there are no ideas separate from material reality*"; that is, human relationships grounded in the sensory activities of daily life are the sites of interest and meaning.

Miriam's childhood was unforgettably unhappy, and like so many of the older people I talked to she'll go to some lengths not to dwell on it. But she knows now that learning how to survive at home with a critical, overbearing sister, a harried and miserable mother, and an oblivious father trained her in an exquisite "attentiveness to the person. So that now, *because I know I remember in a sensory way I never have to say I forget.* Seeing into, sensing something about what people are really doing ... what they are feeling ... how people's emotions make meaning. That is what people remember and talk about." She and Meyer still take classes in sensory awareness on the island in summer, and sometimes in New York in winter—if the weather is not too bad and they can get out or someone drives them. They keep on training their awareness to help them to stay focused on what is most important to them now.

For Miriam, the process is one of continuous observation, a skill she learned so early that it took old age for her to acknowledge that it wasn't automatic, but a product of "the conditions she was born into." Now, discussion and conversation "fasten the facts and bring out memory"—of what interests her, of what she wants to remember. That's why good conversation is so important and one of the reasons that looking after Meyer—passionate as he is about the exchange of ideas—has always been her chief homemaking/life task. She tells me that listening to people, observing them carefully, just as she did as a child with her sister and parents, is how she gets a sense of the person. She can immediately recognize someone's voice on the phone; she gets an image, hears the voice, and sees the person. She can hear strengths and weaknesses, the mood, the excesses.

"When I hear my own voice I think it must be sad, it has such a low pitch."

"Is it? Are you sad?" I ask her.

"No," she replies, "it's more that I'm quieter than Meyer, maybe because he's more moody and demanding. Don't get me wrong, I appreciate the way he thinks. I appreciate that he's still thinking! It's good for us both. But I find more and more that I'm ... that I need to be more low-key."

"Mmm. Could it be that your vital energies have been challenged with your stroke, and so you need to conserve what you have left?"

"Maybe. I don't get distracted—I don't like that word. I can still choose, you know."

"That seems pretty clear! What I've been wondering is, for Martha, working with feelings about her past is still a part of her self-development. And it gives her satisfaction. Even a certain kind of 'pleasure in seeing' as Meyer would say."

"I've done that, I don't need to do it anymore. Most of the time I feel OK about all of that, about who I am."

"More settled in yourself, now that you're older?"

"You could say that."

I told her about my mother's old friend Beatrice. For her, remembering her past is one of her biggest pleasures in the nursing home because there's no one to talk to and she gets really bored. Miriam can see why reminiscence would be satisfying for her, would fill a need, as Meyer would say. But she says she would want to be pretty selective, and she's not sure she can do that.

"Once you get going reminiscing, all sorts of things come up that you don't want to think about. I'm glad I'm not in a place like that, that I'm well enough that with a little help we can still manage on our own."

"What gives you pleasure now?"

"For me, at the end of a day, feeling good is enough."

Afterwards

Meyer died of an embolism a few years after our conversations, and Miriam of a sudden heart attack a year later. I'm glad she went like that. That she didn't linger too long, bored and lonely without Meyer. But I'd like to have had the chance to tell her, now that I'm older and maybe even a little wiser, how feeling good at the end of the day, even with the aches and the limitations, is indeed a pleasure.

"Not enough for you, though," I can hear her say, as she had before.

"No?"

"No. You're just like Meyer. You go after things like a dog with a bone, just like he does. Questioning, questioning, always questioning. And pulling things together. You like that."

"You're right. I do. But you'll always remind me that feeling good is pretty wonderful too."

"You want to have your cake and eat it too."

"I guess. Did you ever hear the saying: 'Too much of a good thing can be wonderful'?"

"Well, I've had all that in my day. But I don't need it now."

I wish.

Simple Pleasures

I love my morning coffee, hedge roses waking
under the sun, the sound of hiker's boots
mud-sliding where the trail begins, rocks
scatter,

voices grumble, kids chatter on the
Schoolhouse steps,
as a golf cart carries the teacher over the rocks
to the door. I watch gulls

swoop over stern-wakes, screaming for entrails
tossed overboard, walk down the road
to the old grey fish house, choose
two from still-bright eyes and shiny scales. Off

to the post office, catch up on the news, read
the notices and gossip on the way
to lobster rolls and Indian Pudding for lunch.
Wait 'til the ferry

nudges to port with the day's trippers.
High-backed rockers on the verandah hide
my eyes closed for "forty winks." New bread,

the earthy smell of fresh vegetables from the
garden,
dinner by the golden glow of the kerosene
lamp,
friends murmuring, piano music drifting

as the sun sets on red velvet rocks.

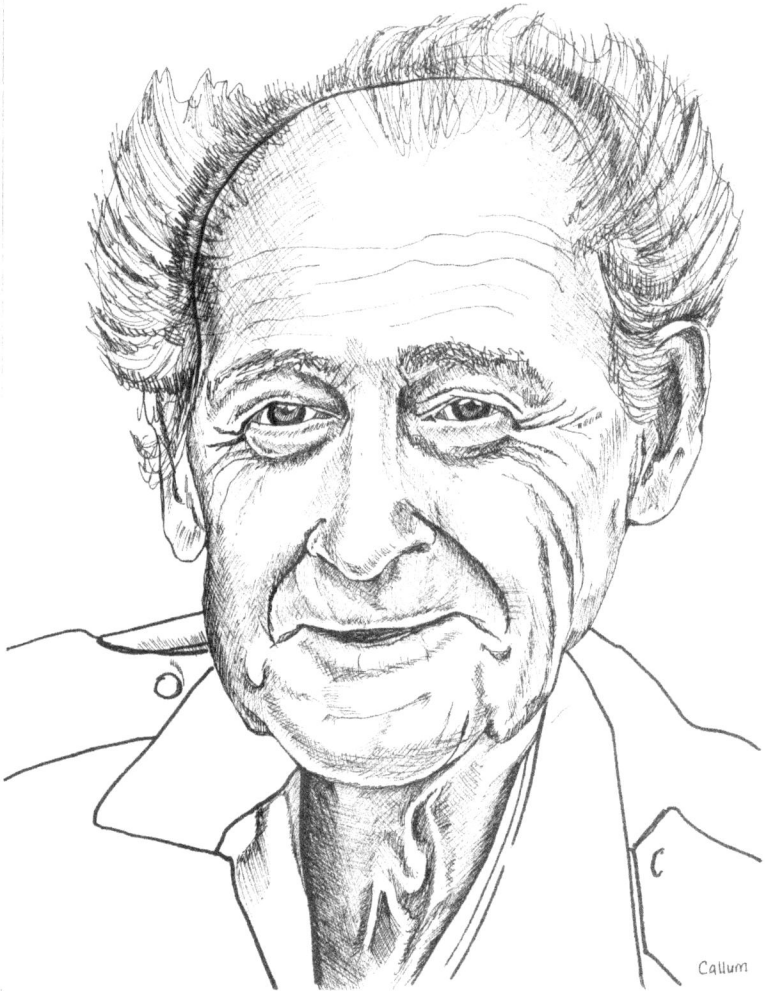

Why Should There Be Thoughts? Callum's Story

"The sensory is the foundation of experience and memory and you cannot talk yourself out of that."

Dressed always in khaki, the colour of his hair, I can see Callum as part of the Mexican sand (where he and Claudia taught in the winter) in the same way that he merges with the colour of the island's dirt road as he makes his way to the post office or grocery store—sites of forgetting—or accompanies Claudia, holding her arm, head tilted to the right in conversation. Slim and short, he moves economically, and his wide blue eyes meet mine directly when we speak, often with a mischievous twinkle when he thinks we are "getting too solemn about serious topics." I sense consideration and immediacy and will always have an image of vitality and spareness when I think about him.

By the time Callum and I talked about memory and aging I had been in the classes he and Claudia taught for three summers, learning sensory awareness as a mindfulness practice that cultivates responsiveness to where we are in the moment, exploring what happens in the simplest of activities, such as breathing, sitting, standing, and walking. The work had alerted me to what I had been calling "body memory," as some of the psychotherapy literature did. I would like to have talked to them both about memory and aging, but Claudia demurred, saying that she disliked writing and talking about her work. Callum agreed and for several afternoons we met on the verandah, or in the sunny front room of their summer home overlooking the harbour, the gulls wheeling around the fishing boats as they returned with the day's catch.

Exploring Memory
Memory and Paying Attention

We talked first about memory, and I was particularly interested to hear his views about the physical sensations that often evoked unnamed emotions and unfamiliar thoughts for me in their classes. He began "at the beginning" with direct sensory experience, next explained how sensory experience becomes a memory, then talked about the process of remembering those experiences, and finally about various ways to express them—"if you have a need to or find you want to."

Direct sensory experience, he explains, is "simply the function of being awake and paying attention. It is not *about* anything, it has nothing to do with thoughts or words. It is immediate sensation," which in itself has nothing to do with memory, but is the foundation of all memory.

He tells me he is aware of this sensory, non-conceptual reality in his life "all the time. When I am cold, I step out in the sunshine. I like it. Simple. It isn't my mind that likes it. It isn't my body that likes it. It is *I* that likes it. And there isn't any verbal element in it; when I walk on grass, words do not occur to me. I just feel it. Right now I feel my feet in my shoes differently than when I walk on grass in my bare feet. Both are clear sensory experiences involving the immediate sensation of having socks and shoes, or not. That is here and now, not memory, as are all moments of pleasure—or pain, like hitting my thumb with a hammer, which I do all too frequently." (During the Second World War Callum was a ship's fitter and went to New York after the war where he became a carpenter and furniture designer.)

A sensory experience becomes a memory "in the moment," he continues, when it has enough emotional or sensory value to make an immediate impression and grab your attention, like the pleasure of walking on grass in his bare feet, quite different from "sentimental or contrived emotion—that is, thinking about how you *ought* to feel." Sensory memories are not indiscriminate or all-inclusive but are those to which we give our attention, filtered through certain criteria. For example, music has very complicated tonal and rhythmic relationships, some of which are immediately appealing to him, some not. The same with colour relationships in painting. "I have never had any trouble in remembering painting and music that has really impressed me." (Similarly, when Meyer and I talked, he observed that sounds have distinct personalities. Emma reported: "Sounds have enjoyment. I suppose it's love, a form of love I feel all through me, which has me remembering." Alice spoke of remembering in pictures: "I make an impression of the whole thing, an association with the form of the whole picture—that you see in terms of your own experience, of course.")

Callum tells me that he is not as open now to taking in new music as he was when he was younger: the "forms, the rhythms and harmonies don't make an immediate impression" and call for a "readjustment to my approach, to my way of listening." (As Alice did after art school.) "My tastes were formed in a certain time." It's much easier for him now to reject art and musical forms that are not "original."

I ask him if, by original, he means recognizable melodies and patterns (thinking of memory as contextual), and he replies, "No, not necessarily." It must be music that catches his attention, and he doesn't waste his time trying to like music that he doesn't want to listen to, such as sentimentally familiar, "tear-jerk stuff," or music that doesn't sound to him as if it has been "felt through. I have eliminated the junk—in literature as well—that which has no emotional or sensory value for me, but is essentially repetitive and boring."

At first I thought that he was rejecting what is new and clinging to the known (which is a cliché in some of the research, and much of the popular thinking, about memory and aging). Thinking about the paradox—that he remembers what he knows, and rejects the familiar—alerts me to the sensory quality of "know," and it dawns on me that he is not rejecting the new in favour of the known. He is rejecting that which is not "original," that is, what is not grounded in concrete, direct sensory experience, or a "new constellation or patterning" of the sensory/experiential. "There is nothing completely new," he comments; "there are only new constellations of things." I ask him what he means, and he jumps up, turns around so his back is to the harbour, and says, "Try looking at it this way," giving me a new perspective on a familiar scene.

The memory literature often reports that we tend to remember what is familiar or known through repetition and rehearsal. Yet according to Callum (and Meyer and Miriam and Russell and Lev), the familiar in the sense of what we learn by rote and is "not felt through"—is too boring to be memorable.

Thinking about the difficulties of paying attention, I tell Callum about an experience I'd had doing Tai Chi, when I was so absorbed watching the fog in the sunlit trees that I stumbled and hurt myself, and he comments: "You were drawn to your surroundings, you did not pay attention to what you were doing. You were somewhere else, not here [touching his chest]. Moment-to-moment attention, that's all that is necessary."

All! At the time it seems huge to me, as I realize for the first time how hard it is for me to *choose* in the here and now among competing "criteria" for my attention. Callum says comfortingly that such confusion and dulled awareness is "the usual case." Nevertheless this experience, and our conversations, were key to my deciding to explore the different worlds of sensory memory.

How we remember sensory experience also involves sensations and feelings: "I remember walking on grass—I can't help but recognize it—and feel now I am not, and it would be more enjoyable if I were."

I ask him if he means that the body remembers in a non-verbal kind of way, and he looks at me quizzically, and asks me why I refer to the body. "*I* remember pleasure and pain. I don't think my body is remembering feeling pleasure or pain. I am."

"You won't feel the rock or the grass and think, 'I am walking on grass, I like it'?"

"No, it's here and now. *Why should there be thoughts?* I think that's what Allan Watts called trying 'to put legs on a snake.'"

He wouldn't think. For me, no-thoughts hover on the verge of no-reality, having been brought up with cogito ergo sum. I ask him, "Who then is the 'I'?" and he replies, "Ah, that is the great unknowable mystery."

Earlier, in a class, I had experienced for the first time in my life a disquieting, "unnameable" sensory memory and so I persisted, "I understand that we are more than our bodies, but when I recall the sensory, isn't that my body remembering?"

"No, I don't think I am more than my body. We are getting into semantics, but we cannot avoid it."

"In the sense that you cannot separate body, mind, and soul?"

"Then why do you speak of memory in the body?" asks Callum.

"I suppose because I haven't found a way of talking about it that gets at non-verbal ways of remembering," I reply.

"When you speak to me that way, you identify yourself with your thought processes. Perhaps it's your university that wants you to encapsulate, perhaps it can't be explained, but do *you* want to?"

"Oh, yes, very much."

"Why else then?" said Callum.

Unravelling How We Remember Sensory Experience

This was a question I couldn't answer then, but it echoed down the years in my wrestling with the patience I needed to recognize my sensory experience—experiences that have never been "first for me"—and then to begin to explore the interleaving depths and layers of sensory memory that seemed so simple to Callum.

He tells me that he can remember tastes and smells that

go way back 70 years to his early childhood, but that he cannot often really identify them—that is, give them a name.

"But you remember them?"

"I do."

"How do you do that?"

"I'm not a neurologist [*a bit sarcastically*]. I would guess that it's an impression on my memory cells that are still in my possession."

"I was thinking of your own experiencing of it."

"Oftentimes I don't remember the circumstances. A smell will be familiar, but when and where ... sometimes that will come."

Then we come to *expressing sensory memories and experiences,* and that is difficult. We can recognize them when we are alert to them, but to name or explain them in what (for Callum's friend Russell) is the "usual way"—that is, logically and rationally—is another matter, as I was just then realizing (although, as Callum pointed out, neurologists have their theories). However, he believes that we *can* intuitively share sensory experiences without needing to talk about them, although we may not be aware that we're doing so.

"My sensory experience is so obviously related to certain situations. I could say, 'Isn't it a nice sunny day?' and you'd say, 'Oh, isn't it.' Essentially it just means that we have shared an experience that's very common. There's no such thing as a completely shared experience, although much is shared partially. We might just smile at each other."

Smile lines crinkling around his eyes remind me that we share without saying a word in his classes. We can spend an entire morning exploring the weight and feel of an arm at rest and in motion, on our own, or moved slowly by a partner; and then the afternoon walking the island trails in an intense, concentrated, wordless practice of being with our physical selves in the moment ... deeper than mind awareness.

I ask him now how he would attempt to talk about what happened in class. He says that in the first place he isn't sure he could actually tell anybody, although, while much of it is unknowable, he might be able to share some aspect of it: "I think we can intuitively feel what I'm getting across, a sense of moving together, when it's really matching, like dance [calypso dance and percussion are lifelong interests] or like all intimate relations when they are functioning freely—but how often is that?" (Shades of Meyer.)

Music and painting, he tells me, express the sensory when they too are "functioning freely"—that is, when they are "felt through," and communicate the artist's sensory and emotional consciousness and experiences.

"It is not essential to *describe* an experience in order to have the memory of it—consciousness isn't necessarily verbal. Only if you are a writer and want to communicate in that way are words necessary." And when it comes to words, Callum thought that only poets truly express sensory experience. Even then, all words are merely symbols, abstract and removed from experience; "the great unknowable mystery" can't really be put into words.

"I reject a great many words," he states firmly.

"But words are so ever-present in our lives," I blurt out. "It's hard to do without them."

"How pervasive is the value placed on words. I doubt my very existence when I have no words for her, remember my mother telling me to 'use my words,' that only when I could express myself in words could I be understood. I keep on insisting that somehow my body should BE words, that memories be located in mind-words" (My Grandmother's Hair, Edgar Kent, 2006, p. 155).

He knows this. As if reading my mind, he adds, "I feel that the enemy of direct experience is our tendency to verbalize, which occupies consciousness, which is therefore not open to the message of the sensory. People haven't grown up being fully aware of their own experience, and often haven't been permitted to speak about their experiences. We are not interested in the real child."

The universe, he points out, is relative, and that is what modern science is all about. Sensory or experiential reality is relational, as are music, art—and mathematics. "I have a great respect for mathematics as the study of processes; it is much closer to the experiential because it is about relationships. The basis of mathematics is the difference between this and this"— he holds up one finger of one hand and two of the other— "which isn't the difference between words. This is much closer to experience. There are no absolutes in experience, or mathematics, there is no fast or slow, only faster or slower."

Finding Words, "if you have a need to or want to."

When he does "remember the circumstances," Callum can bring his sensory and emotional experience "to mind and find words for it, but at the time it happened, it was no *memory* of experience." A writer looking for appropriate words for past experience must recall and remember and at the same time choose "from the stock of words in memory those which fit together to describe the experience."

Callum informs me that he had written a manuscript describing in great detail the experience of a day or two. Meyer was amazed and told him he must have total recall.

"I was able to relive those experiences very fully. So much so that whether they were interesting to other people or not, they did seem real. I did something like that years ago, in 1963, and hope to try it again in the next year or so. When I do, it will be a lot easier for me to give some answers to whether or not my memory has changed over time. I do know I want to, whether in my present way of living I can take out the time I would need to do it … We are living in different circumstances now; soon I will be going abroad to teach there with Claudia. We will have time there, but not the place." It would be easy for him to write this book on the island, because it is the right kind of place (to which I can attest—I began to write poetry again when I was there). If they could stay on the island for six months, he would probably attempt it.

And I wonder, with Callum, whether it's possible to become fully aware of sensory experience as an adult if you've not been allowed to be fully aware of your physical and emotional being as a child.

"We all have quite a memory of words, a large or small vocabulary that is entirely different from sensory experience, from any experience," he continues. "The verbal is symbolic in the same way that mathematics learned by rote is. And a symbol is *not* a memory of experience; it is something eventually associated with somebody else's experience."

Pots and pans memory

Callum can remember long Latin quotes that he learned on his own, out of interest, rather than in school. This kind of memory is different again from what he calls "pots and pans" memory. He has no trouble remembering where something is in the kitchen—if it is where he put it and someone hasn't misplaced it, or with any of the other "ordinary mechanisms of daily life." Then there is what he calls making "mental notes"— the kind of thought process he uses when he reminds himself to look at the calendar to remember that he was going to do something on a particular day, or to make lists for packing or shopping.

As for names, he remembers only those with an emotional association—such as mine, because he was annoyed that he had agreed to an appointment with me! Otherwise he forgets names and thinks that's because he sees many people over the course of a year, not because of aging.

Not remembering names hasn't been nearly as worrisome to him as the way he has "fallen into the habit" of forgetting objects that he carries around and then sets down. When he recalls his "habit of forgetting," he will "take action," perhaps smacking the table and saying, "I'm laying it here!"

"A way of getting your attention?" I ask.

"Exactly," he replies, "because I am often ambivalent about what I should remember."

He thinks this stance is "a complicated psychological attitude about the whole process of doing things. I don't know what Freud would say about it, although I would be the first to consult him if we could bring him back, but I do feel it would be profitable if I were to work on this memory problem."

He offers other examples of how his ambivalence affects his memory. He does most of the shopping and cooking (which he didn't do in his first marriage), which he says has its pluses and minuses. Partly he likes doing it, partly he resents doing it, and so he'll forget to make a list and then not remember what he is supposed to buy, "which is a great nuisance, because it's a long trip back to the house." When he enters the store he has the sensation that his mind is blocking out certain things. He doesn't "have a system," such as looking at the signs, as Rivka does. Often something will trigger his memory. "Let's say I see a mop standing, and then I say, 'Oh, yes, I want some powdered soap.' Really, I function so much better when I make a list, but I usually don't. I don't have an intelligence in simple systems, simply a place to write down the errands. Some people do, but I haven't. If I haven't made a list—which does seem to depend on my state of mind when I set out—I think I have a little feeling of 'To hell with it, life will go along one way or another without it.' And I want to get done with it and get back to where I came from."

"A state of feeling, not thinking?" I ask.

"I don't make a distinction between the two," he replies.

Aspects of Aging
Aging and Maturity

"Frankly, I call it immaturity," Callum comments about his lack of a "simple system." "I think I do it less than I did 30 years ago. I haven't as much energy as I had then, and I may feel more ambivalent about shopping and doing all these things that are really self-imposed tasks." He also calls it laziness and feels slovenly and careless. When I comment on how he seems judgmental about himself, he replies, "Very true. That's why I call it immature. I feel I ought to have outgrown that kind of judging of myself."

Forgetting to pack something when he's going on a trip is the same kind of thing: he feels very anxious before starting off, even more so when he and Claudia are going together. He's sure they have forgotten something, "and we usually have. The reason? I call it inertia. The ambivalence about going anywhere rather than just staying where I am sets off an emotional conflict: 'I want to go, I don't want to go.' 'I don't want to go' expresses itself in a sense of anxiety that is very strong and often makes me very disagreeable.

"In my woodworking shop, in painting the house, I have a very strong disinclination to put things away after I've used them. I do imagine that it's because of my own mother's anxiety when I was little about things being put away and her making a moral issue of it."

"That's connected to those judgments you make about yourself?"

"I don't doubt that," Callum replies. "And this again is immaturity. Failure to grow out of my childhood into full maturity. Ambivalence about going back to my childhood. I see maturity as a very simple process of not losing the good aspects of childhood while realizing that childish conditions no longer prevail. I haven't accepted myself as fully as I think would be appropriate. My mother's been dead for 20 years."

"And she's still speaking to you."

"I think she is! And the worst thing is, she's speaking in non-verbal terms."

"How does she do that?"

"Her own anxiety."

"A transmission of feeling?"

"Yes, the feeling that goes with an obligation to do something. Not for the obvious reason that makes it worth doing, like wearing a carpenter's apron so I don't lose my hammer by forgetting where I put it down, but for some vague moral reason—if someone says this is right, and something else, something I'm doing, or not doing, is wrong. My guess is it must be true of a great many others as they grow up."

I ask him if that is what he meant when he said that we are not interested in the real child and tell him that Meyer feels much the same way. He replies that he and Meyer often think along the same lines. One of the reasons he loves teaching sensory awareness is that he has learned not to project his needs on his students (the way his mother did to him) and to be more in tune with *their* needs, and so he has become a much better teacher over the years.

"Is it easier to tune in to someone's needs in a sensory way, rather than verbally, through questions and so forth?"

"Oh, yes, that's what relationships are all about."

For Callum, aging involves bringing the unconscious to consciousness, so that as he ages he can "have [both] his experience and now the observation of it" without self-judgment. When I say that for me this also means bringing the sensory to awareness, he agrees. This is part of the "pluses and minuses" of the process, since remembering the good aspects of childhood means somehow convincing himself that not all of "the conditions of childhood prevailed"—that he no longer has to listen to his mother's voice.

"A kind of forgetting," I say.

"Yes, if you like. And it's difficult, because it's sensory."

"A sensory experience is harder to forget?"

"Oh, yes, especially when it happens before we learn words."

He might "curse and swear" when his ambivalence about the "whole process of doing things" induces forgetfulness, but he is calm about his immaturity. It is clear, that for him, maturing is a lifelong process and that he regards himself as very much in that process, as in: "I am sure it would be profitable for me to work on that problem," and his wry, "Whether or not I will is another question; it depends very much on my current circumstances." "Circumstances" being his elliptical way of alluding to his sensory, mental, and social "conditions," which are inseparable.

Dimensions of Aging

Like many of the people I talked to, Callum does the same sorts of things as he did when he was younger. He still has a zest for life—enjoys teaching, cooking, gardening—but finds himself more limited: he still takes long walks but can't run up hills anymore; he used to dance with several groups every week, but now does circle dancing once a week. However, it's easier for him to accept or reject what he likes and dislikes, because he has clearer criteria and priorities (as he mentioned in connection with music and painting). One of the advantages of aging: a lifetime in literature and the arts, and in teaching and working with his hands, has enlarged his experience so that he "now has a better store of useful memories at my disposal than I did earlier, and a great deal of that experience is still available to me, which is my only hope for writing a book."

The downside: "The number of significant books has multiplied enormously, and I'm just not anywhere equal to it." He is keen to keep up with world information, but it's difficult to decide what would be "reasonable and sensible of me to read. I don't know whether to attribute that to having less energy as I get older, or to becoming less self-involved than I was years ago, and being more open to the difficult world situation, about which there is so much intelligent information these days. It's not possible for me not to want to make these discriminations."

When I inquire about changes in the way he remembers in the previous 30 or 40 years, or in the strategies he uses, he doesn't think there are many changes, and doesn't think of using strategies—"although trying to remember the groceries could be a strategy, I suppose." How would he talk to others about his experience of memory? He'd like to find the words, but "nothing comes to me. I don't really think about it, it's simply an experience."

Not finding words to describe his remembering and forgetting doesn't bother Callum at all, but it does bother me, as he notes, and queries. When he wonders why I am trying to explain sensory memory, he comments that for him academic pursuits are the "embodiment of the human tendency to petrify things … the whole idea of absolute divisions in contradiction to the universe, where everything is relative." Moreover, he tells me, he doesn't think my project belongs in the academic world, and he was right, as I was to discover much later.

Different Viewpoints

In thinking about our conversations, and in trying to find words for his views and experience of sensory memory that will make some kind of sense to the general reader, I began to see that it is my struggle to find words and explanations that draws my attention to my own sensory world. This is not so for him. He inhabits a different world, where thinking and words are not always necessary.

I tell him of an experience I'd had going to the hospital for a minor procedure. I felt far more anxious than was warranted and puzzled over the reason, finally remembering a former, traumatic hospital experience that might have been the cause.

"I was aware of an intense feeling of anxiety in my body."

"Where else would it be?" he asks.

"I was not able to put the anxiety and the pain together with any name."

"So, by your body, you mean your unconscious mind?" He's puzzled.

"No, it was a physical sensation. I wasn't thinking anxiety, I felt a nameless sensation."

"But anxiety isn't verbal, it's an emotion."

"But I couldn't say, 'This is anxiety.' All I could say was that I had pain. I couldn't link it to anything, and the closer I got to the hospital the worse it got. I had forgotten in my head those other operations. Afterwards, when it finally came to me, I had a sense that my body knew far better than I did."

"When you speak to me this way, you are identifying

yourself with your thought processes again. Perhaps as far as academic work is, you have to. Your speaking to me of body memory throws things out of gear."

"What would you say?"

"I call it my memory."

"I am aware of trying to explain something that is almost inexplicable."

"Maybe it can't be explained."

Here I sense a flutter of panic. He is so calm. Not to be able to explain? How can I know? For me, knowledge has always been of the mind, in thinking. He is suggesting that knowledge can be somewhere else ... I have never found any other place ... and HE has never found a place for grocery lists. He doesn't seem to be a linear person, or to be very concerned about it.

"Perhaps it can be given pictorial form?" I ask.

"Yes, I think so. That's the function of art, conveying non-conceptual reality. And many memories are just that."

The Roots of Memory

Callum's assertion that direct sensory experience is the foundation of memory is not a new idea. This concept is the basis of the information-processing model of memory, although it is not often elaborated in terms of individual sensory experiences, other than in terms of deficits such as loss of hearing and vision. Nor do researchers usually explore the social production of sensory experience in our environment from our earliest years, through school, jobs, and retirement, and in cultural concepts of the self and attitudes about youth and old age.

For Callum, the sensory is experience, is a non-conceptual reality. He talks about the cognitive as if it is conceptual only and not experiential. His insistence that the sensory cannot be conceptual, because it does not involve thoughts, polarized him as identifying with the sensory, just as Russell's and Lev's conviction that memory is solely cognitive identified them with the cognitive at the expense of recognizing the power of the sensory in memory.

But to hear the way Callum talks about what sensory memory *is*, was new to me. Coming from so intellectual a background, I did not grow up with a "consciousness of the sensory," and I was in awe of the "childish conditions" that permitted Callum to do so. At first I assumed, based on my own yearning, that his "original," direct sensory experiences were positive ones. I was drawn in with his speaking of the innocence and joy of the non-verbal sensory, as if only the verbal and cognitive bring pain. At first I ignored what the childish conditions might be that he wished to leave behind. But when he talked about ambivalence and forgetting and the anxiety that his mother's voice evoked, I realized that many of his sensory experiences were painful for him. I had been lured on the thread of my own desire into thinking he could forget them.

Seeing this (as Meyer would say), I noticed several absences in our interviews. Like my conversations with Meyer, mine with Callum was predominantly theoretical, and there were even fewer specific, concrete examples of his direct sensory experience, sensory remembering, or sensory memories. His somewhat distant references to pain, as in "disagreeable," "uncomfortable," and "nuisance," highlighted for me the fact that my incomprehension about sensory memory related to my reluctance to allow pain, shame, and fear as "sense perception of forms," forms of relationships that I too wanted to leave behind. He was sure that my anxiety could be nowhere else but "in the body," but he did not mention how or where he felt the anxiety evoked by his mother's voice, and did not mention pain as having sensory and emotional value for him until we discussed forgetting.

Looking for Clues about Callum

Remembering what so many of the people I talked to had said about not wanting to remember past hurts and pain, and

Meyer's conviction that such emotions were a kind of baggage that was a "barrier to understanding," I wondered about other aspects of Callum's life that he had to keep on reminding himself no longer prevailed. Because of my own recently remembered sensory experiences, which I wrote about in *My Grandmother's Hair*, I was alert to possible examples of how the dominance of the cognitive can oppress the physical. Where was sensory language as a means of social construction in his discourse on memory? Where is the sensory language of discomfort that shaped him?

I knew so very little of his past, despite having known him for many years. I knew him in the here and now: knew the sensitive teacher, had tasted his excellent fish soup when he invited our class to dinner and seen the pleasure he took in our enjoyment, and had admired the garden that was his pride and joy, which he had expertly landscaped in harmony with the rocky Maine terrain (different to the one in California, he eagerly explained, when I inquired), and the simple, beautifully finished furniture he'd made for their house. I had rocked with laughter at the stories he told after dinner, watched the play of emotions on his face as he listened to the island concerts. He had told me how much he missed dancing and hiking. I had read about his father—historian, biographer, and literary critic—whom other people had told me had "driven his wife and sons almost crazy" moving the family all over Europe and the United States to accommodate his teaching schedule and lecture circuit. I could guess a little about that relationship in Callum's quiet pride in being able to describe his "sensations and feelings as if they were real—even though they might not interest other people." (Even his wordsmith father?)

After he died, I read about the facts of his life and the heartfelt affection of his friends in the memorial and tributes offered at the funeral. Only when I came on the opening pages of the memoirs he began and so wanted to finish before he died, reprinted in another newsletter, did I gain a few clues about the questions that haunted me about the "childish conditions" that had shaped his life and formed his theory of sensory experience and memory. He wrote that he was "orientated to water ... Life is like 10,000 lakes only mine are mostly salt ... originating with my mother, carried through her memory to me before I was born. Her fear of water ... great was her fear and great her courage." He had his own "rite of passage with water: I filled a deep tub, locked the door and lay down in the bone-chilling water, determined to stay until I could accept it. After a few minutes somebody knocked at the door. I called, 'I'll be out soon,' and the person left. Very slowly the sense of cold grew less. I became peaceful, then drowsy. On the verge of falling asleep I realized that if I did, I might not awaken. Did it matter? It did. I struggled out, with great difficulty dried myself and managed to return to my room. There was a hot radiator. Covering it with a towel, I pressed against it and for perhaps an hour shook uncontrollably." That was all he wrote—relived fully so that he "described it as if it were real."

Where is the line—is there a line?—between direct experience and the story of our existence?

As If It Were Real: Callum's Poem

When the radio in the mind is stilled, everything else can come to life. The camper's lantern is blown out and the darkness fills with stars as the woods deepen and widen. The primitive world in which things appear and disappear, bloom and fade, eat and are eaten surrounds us and includes us. We cannot know the future, and only the least trace of the past. But when we breathe in the air of the night woods, and let their forms and almost imperceptible worlds into us ... and perhaps feel the earth sustaining us, we know that we exist, at first hand, surrounded by innumerable other beings who exist too. Need we ask more?

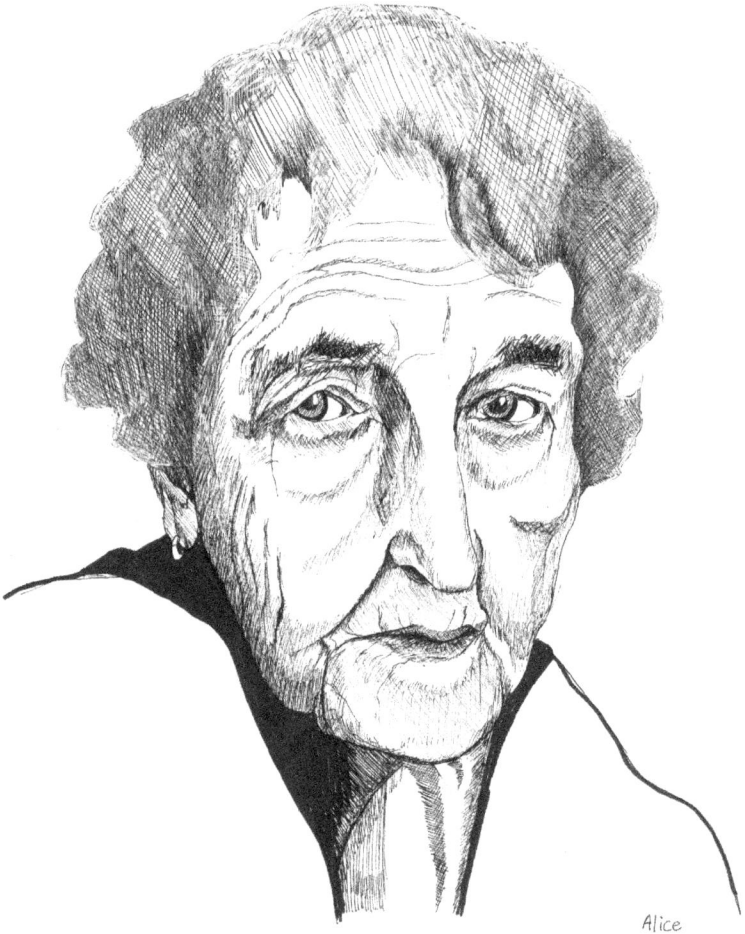

Alice

Living Your Passion: Alice's Story

"Keep on doing what you love to do."

Walking up the hill from the boat I see that Alice is there again, a thin little figure in blue, perched on a stool in front of her easel on the lawn of the inn, three storeys of New England white frame with green trim rising behind her, ladder-backed rocking chairs on the wraparound verandah waiting for day trippers to have their after-lunch coffee. With her art supplies to one side on the grass, sporting a big floppy hat that hides her face, except for the determined jut of her chin, she concentrates on her painting. The way she sits, upright, the way she works without pause, you would never guess that she turned 89 that year. After seeing my bags onto the truck that would take them to my temporary home on the island, I walk farther up the dirt road and across the lawn to where she sits. She pulls back to look at her work, stretches, and then spots me, hesitating a little. I can see she has forgotten my name, and then she smiles, remembering.

"You're a writer aren't you? I remember we talked about memory and getting old."

"That's right, I'm Ann Carson. You haven't changed a bit in two years, Alice. How are you?"

"I'm just fine. At my age, one more wrinkle doesn't make a lot of difference! You look well, too. How long will you be here?"

"For three wonderful weeks, and you?"

"Almost that. I got here two days ago, been painting ever since."

"Do you think you'll have time for us to get together?"

"Oh, I think so. When Rob told me you were coming this year, I remembered you'd mentioned it before. But in the evening, after I've done all that I want to do, and after supper."

"Of course. That's wonderful, whenever you'd like— just let me know."

A Show of Her Own!

I settle in at my room in the hostel. Walk a few of my favourite trails out to the high side of the island. I need a few days sitting on rocks looking out over the ocean curving away to the horizon, my skin thirsty for the salt spray mist thrown up by waves crashing on the rocks below. When I finally feel at home again, and she has time, I meet Alice after dinner in the lounge at the inn. We don't sit in the big chintz chairs by the fire but find a place in one of the little alcoves looking out on the harbour, where we can be by ourselves.

Alice can hardly wait to tell me that after all the years of small shows, or being in group shows—"I was always 'one of,' you know. One of a group of American women artists, or pioneer artists, or early watercolourists. That sort of thing"— she had won a solo show in May and a cash prize as well. And then in November, after she'd been to the island she'd put one of the summer's watercolours into the National Arts Club Show and won $100 and a $150 frame—to use in the January exhibition—for a canvas that she'd done on her very first visit to the island in 1934, of the same dock, only from a different position. She leans forward, tipping her head towards the harbour down the hill.

"You can see it way over there now ... the first award ever given for a painting done 53 years ago. The other award was for a painting I did last summer, from near the entrance, looking down at the sunset, which was simply glorious. It was just one of those times it was simply magnanimous—I mean 'magnificent,' not 'magnanimous'—but I guess that's how it felt, as if nature was just so generous."

"She so often is up here—I remember the northern lights that sang, do you?"

"Oh, yes, I do. When we all sat on the fire-escape stairs for hours and had to make hot tea around midnight to warm up."

"You've been painting for a long time."

"All my life."

"Do you remember when you began?"

Childhood Loss

Leaning back in her chair, she tells me that she started to draw when she was four years old and made Christmas presents for the family. Her Aunt Edith did exquisite hand-painted china, flowers on plates with gold leaf. Alice used to watch the way she held her hand, and then one day she found a stone along the beach and decided to paint it for her father. Her aunt gave her paints and a brush, and she made a sailboat on the water that her father kept until he died.

"Ahh—that's lovely."

"Mmm. All the women in my family were talented in the arts of homemaking. My mother made beautiful quilts, my other aunt did marvellous tatting, my grandmother made delicious pies. She was a marvellous cook."

They grew their own vegetables, kept chickens, and bought barrels of flour because they were a long way out of town, with no stores nearby. Alice remembers her aunt putting a stick in some earth, and in a few weeks it started to grow, and so she stuck one in too … and that became a grape arbour, by the time she was 16 or 17.

"I've had a very happy life—I had a very nice childhood overall." She looks away for a while, turns back with a small smile: "But sad. I lost a brother and sister in the wintertime when I was four-and-a-half years old."

"I'm sorry. How did that happen? That was awful, two children at the same time."

"Out there in the flatlands—Flatbush, Brooklyn, New York—the old Dutch section, you know. And, of course, malignant scarlet fever was what it was, and they had no antibiotics for it then—and so for a long time … My youngest sister was born after that, and she was our little ray of sunshine, you know, and my one brother was left. He was five years older, and so I was in-between. It's a strange thing, you have to be resourceful and work on your own ideas when you're in-between."

"'Cause you're right in the middle."

"Uhuh … yes, in the middle. But they …" she veers away from speaking that particular thought and goes on to tell me that she had a very loving mother and father. Because they were so isolated, her father helped around the house—not so usual in those days. They stayed way out in Flatbush until Alice was seven-and-a-half and then moved up to Rugby Road, where she went to a public grammar school—No. 139—for the first time. She'd learned a lot at home and didn't think much of school until she went to high school and took drawing classes all four years, as well as the academic requirements. Her instructors encouraged her to go to art school, and her father agreed when she won a scholarship for three years and didn't have to pay tuition.

Acceptance by the Pratt Institute—"one of the best"—pleased her, and the instruction there continued with what she had started in high school—"a way of seeing. This wonderful teacher I had used to say that if you were going someplace and you saw something, like out of the window of a bus or a trolley, as soon as you can you must make a note to see how much you can remember of that, 'cause lots of times you can't go back and see it again. And anyway, even if you did, it wouldn't be the same thing."

Always Composing

The human figure fascinates her, and she loves to watch people, on the bus or whenever she's travelling: "I find everybody sitting there with their hands a certain way, looking right and left, sometimes just sitting. If you catch their eye, because you're studying their faces, and you just smile a little bit, they smile back, and their whole face is different, because the muscles of the face either drop, or go up, and from then on they're interested in you and you have a kind of rapport with their eyes."

She learned a particular way of looking at the world and of how to remember what she saw and tells me that she always sees in pictures. Looking at me, she pauses, cocks her head to one side, and says that she could make a painting of me right then, choosing from the background what she wants, moving a chair or a plant to get the composition just right. "I am always composing."

"Always composing, like putting people and things into relationships?"

"Into little compositions. See, there are six fundamentals involved, and composition is one of them; that's something you learn in art school."

"Do you remember the shapes, or the spaces between, or ...?"

"I remember impressions."

"Impressions. And that's a total thing?"

"Total. Total impression. Of what my memory of it was. My teacher would say: 'Just take along the small things. Even if you want to paint it right there, first of all, see what you can remember.'"

"Lev once told me that when he's remembering something he wants to paint—or even just remembering—the scene unrolls before him like a movie script."

"No, no," Alice is vehement, "it's nothing like a camera, not the *scene*, that's an impression. (Callum would agree.) But your *mind* is almost like a camera, because you're choosing. Because of being an artist, you are choosing your arrangements."

I ask her how she is aware of what she is choosing, and she responds that it almost always has a particular balance, has a movement to it, which is one of the seven motifs, such as lines, circles, and spirals, that they learned in art school, and that when you've been working all your life "your mind knows just what to do."

"You've trained your mind and ..."

"You've trained your mind. I think that's the best way to put it. You've trained your mind how to paint what you see. When I teach, I explain all that."

"So you don't necessarily remember everything, then?"

"Oh, no. You don't want to."

"You don't want to?"

"No, no, you're choosing. It's your choice really ... Now, I have definitely done a very literal drawing of that scene I want to paint. I will put away that drawing entirely if it's a glorious morning tomorrow, and I can get that wonderful effect of the sunrise that only comes for a short time—that's why I'm doing it, in that span of time."

"Another kind of choice?"

"I want to get the same light where the shadows do what I want them to; they come in a beautiful place, the colour is marvellous, and it's just right in relation to—see—I could almost make a small sketch now ... Maybe I will do that ... maybe."

I ask her if she wants to stop so that she can paint what she's visualizing, but she demurs, saying that since she's on the island she'll wait to catch the real thing at the right time: "But if I wasn't here, I could do it—I can see the entire scene."

Earning a Living

The first sitting in the dining room is over—Alice was one of the earliest diners, at 5:30. Many of the summer islanders waiting for the second sitting know Alice and stop by to ask her about her painting. She smiles and chats, introduces me to a few of them, and then, when the last one is through the door into the dining room she turns to me and says how wonderful it is for her to have made painter friends on the island and to have the kind of professional conviviality here that she had known at the Pratt, where they were all learning together.

Especially exciting and interesting for her is doing something she's always loved and to be able to share that with other people.

After art school, she had married "the very man I met the first day, an artist like me" and soon after they had a son. She painted portraits on commission, winning several prizes from W.J. Sloan Interiors in New York, as well as teaching industrial arts for eight years. When her son went off to school, she started her own work, in watercolour—back then, something "suitable for a woman would be china painting and all that, you know. But I had graduated from the Pratt, taught all those years, and my husband liked my work and encouraged me to join the professional associations ..."

As we talk, I'm aware of how alike we are here. Although several generations apart, we both turned a domestic art into a profession: she, decorating china into watercolour painting, and I, caring for my children into psychotherapy, another kind of caring, and later, as she has, into being curious about memory.

"... My son stayed in school for lunch," Alice continued, "so unless they had a day off, or he was sick, I'd have most of the day to myself. I'd hurry to get the chores done so I could get on with my real work."

I told her that Miriam and I had talked about how well-organized you have to be to juggle home and career, that she'd been able to teach after she married because her child died in infancy and the board had to make a place for her, but that she still had all the home responsibilities.

"Of course she did," Alice says, and goes on to say that a woman could teach in art school after she married, even after children came—"if you could manage it all; art schools didn't have the same rules." But she's had to "regiment" herself all her life to manage it all. When she was teaching in Newark, she'd get up at 6 o'clock, straighten up the studio so it looked like a studio—her first apartment in Greenwich Village was one room—get ready, go down ten flights of stairs ...

"Ten flights!" I exclaimed.

"Oh, I was young then. I could get a 35-cent breakfast—egg, toast, and coffee—and then go to Montague Street, take the subway to the city—New York City—and then take the bus up to art school. And be there by a quarter to nine. And that is the same thing I did when I was married and I still do today. Now, I hardly ever can paint early, I'm always better a little later in the day to work."

Finding Your Own Voice

Her mind has to "take it easy for a while." Like Lev, she can't just rush into creative things, has to "let herself into it." When she was younger, she rented a room at the island's hostel and did more or less what she wanted. Now she stays at the inn—"not for as long, because it's much more expensive—and it's hard to be regimented again, with 8 o'clock breakfast and other meals at set times.

"It's noisy, too, with so many people. But I get looked after—it's wonderful, really, to have all my energy for painting, so I can get up early in the morning at 5:30 and do the wonderful sunrise coming up over the rocks first thing. In the two days since I've been here, I've done a painting this size. Here, I want to show you." She reaches down into the bag at her feet and carefully pulls out a canvas. "It's coming along nicely. I feel happy about it."

"I would recognize that right away as an Alice Rowland."

"Really?" She smiles.

"Sure. I knew your paintings long before I met you. I'd see them at the inn and at the Island Gallery. There's something that has always fascinated me: there are many sunrise paintings in the Gallery. How does it happen that I can tell which painting belongs to a particular artist—or that I haven't a clue who's done it because it's just like, well, just another painting?"

"You have to see it in terms of your own experience."

"How do you eliminate the details you don't want until you have the essence of what you *do* want?"

She looks past me into the next room, seems to have gone away for a while, and then come back: "You have to be alone, you have to be off by yourself, your pen and brush lying there." She tells me that some members of the group that work with the same models at the Art Studio League in New York have something of the same technique in all their work, which is natural—they are young and still learning and haven't "got into being confident yet. To come to your own style, you have to get away from school."

"That's just the beginning, school."

"I've made that very clear with everyone I've ever taught. It's very important, and I loved teaching—I still do—but it's just the start."

"It's like a fingerprint, isn't it? Or like the old storytellers who took a traditional story and made it into a song a contemporary audience could understand. How do *you* do that? It's so difficult to put into words. Do you think, for yourself, you can have visual memories that can't be expressed in words, at least not adequately?"

"Yes, I do. What you're seeing may be so elusive that you just can't entirely get it, but you do what you feel is the nearest you can come to it, but you should never have to explain. Your paintings do. If it's good enough to appeal to someone and has caught what you caught and felt deeply when you did it, there's no explanation necessary. If there is, it means that the other person lacks the ability to see."

"So it's a two-way street? The person who 'gets it' speaks the same language in a sense. It's something the same with memory, isn't it? There's a shared language or context, and it's not necessarily words. Often when people talk about memory, you would think that memory has to do only with words."

"It's a two-way street, it has to be. And memory doesn't have just to do with words, because the mind is bigger than words, the mind is immense. We have a marvellous organism of a body that is being controlled—right down to my little finger, even any motion that I'm making—is being controlled by that place up there." *Points to her forehead.*

Alice is astonished that she remembers everything she sees. If she's been to a place once, she knows how to get there again. If she wants to remember it, she draws it. A wonderful teacher of hers said that there are as many ways of painting as there are people in the world.

"And as many ways of remembering as there are people in the world? Meyer says that he made an emotional attachment to music at an early age so that sound became his form of memory. Is finding the impression and painting it your form of memory?"

"Yes, it is. You see, you learn a system of observing, of organizing your mind, which is much more than thinking—because the mind is vast and encompasses impressions, feelings, movement. People learn to remember in different ways, depending on how they've been trained, like Meyer says. See, you have to have a common language: music, art, dance. I don't know what people do if they haven't had any training, any experience of that. Because if there's no common language, there's no communication—and so no memory. You have to communicate in some way for there to be memory, don't you?"

I agreed and ask her if she remembers the guest at the inn who regaled people with her stories of the island. Sharing her stories was her common language. I had marvelled that she could remember the names of people going back 50 years and more. Alice, ever practical, reminds me that her family had owned the inn, then sold it to Rod who had it now. "So, of course she would remember names—that's important for an innkeeper, makes people feel welcome, and then you get them back. Now, I have a bad memory for names. See, I know you've told me your name, but I forget what it is."

"It's Ann—I'm the same way, I forget names but I never forget a face."

"Exactly, remembering the person. But I don't exactly forget the name; I just might not be able to think of it. It will come back to me when I get the association with the form, with the whole picture, probably when I'm going to bed and thinking about our talk in here, the fire, people coming and going in the background, what we can see of the sunset from in here."

Reserving our coveted alcove space with bags and sweaters, we join a few people outside on the porch to watch the sunset. Nobody speaks. I remember that when we gather like this there are never any voices until the sun is completely down and ask Alice later if it was as reminiscent for her of age-old rituals as it was for me. She points out that sunsets are rarely painted, because it's almost impossible to capture that kind of power. "It's an ending. Sunrise is easier, something hopeful about the beginning of a day."

Murmuring quietly among themselves, members of the little gathering move back inside or off up the road to their several houses.

Engaging All the Senses

"Where were we?" Alice asks. "You were saying your memory isn't so much auditory as ... Oh yes, I've had difficulty learning languages. I did a little French and Latin, but it was book learning, the words in a book."

"Not ear learning."

Laughs. "No, not ear learning."

"So how are you with music? Your son is an opera singer."

"Oh, I love music and listen a lot." She may not remember exact tunes, but if it's something she knows, she will remember that it's Chopin or Bach. Her younger sister was a concert pianist and played all the things Alice loved, "so when I'd be painting in the next room, she'd be playing the piano. I remember the whole picture. And when I went to Italy with my son when he was learning opera I learned—I can hear them in my ear—I can hear *Aïda*, the last act. I can hear certain solos he's sung in *Bohème* and *Rigoletto*."

"He's a tenor, then?"

"Yes," *laughing with delight.* "Wonderful operas, I love opera. I've heard so many in rehearsal, that's how I got to remember them. But I only enjoy the real ones, though, not on TV, where you get close-ups of those faces with their mouths wide open and nice white teeth. It takes away the illusion."

"The magic."

"The magic. Well, I think that's the thing an artist tries to create is magic maybe. That's a good word."

"When you describe how you remember a particular scene or an aria or a person or to paint a picture, it's as if you were taking the essence of that."

"That's the important word. That's what I think of, essence, or truth, the character in a person. I look for eyes almost always because for me eyes tell everything. Another friend of mine looks at the mouth."

Alice's saying how she watched her aunt's hand as she painted reminded me that hands are what I look at first. Alice isn't surprised at that and goes on to say that painting hands is important and very difficult, that many artists, when they put their work into exhibitions, do the head and body wonderfully, "but if they have hands and feet, they do clubs. Clubby, clubby, clubby, gross in relation to this exquisite part they have created above—they've only thought of that. But an artist has to think of everything; it isn't just one part, it's the whole. That's another word we use when we speak of art—whole."

"Well, the essence, the whole—" *we say in unison, laughing together.*

I mention that Lev told me he didn't put hands in his paintings because he couldn't paint them well, and I'd wondered if that was because he started out self-taught. She replies, "That could be, you know; you'd feel pretty isolated and wonder about yourself maybe. I don't know that I could have … I've always felt surrounded by artists. I'm sure that's what helped me carry on painting even when I was raising my son and so tired with having to juggle so many things."

This is the first time Alice has mentioned how tired she was trying to be a good housewife and mother and a good artist as well. I can remember not talking about my constant fatigue either, because if I did people would give me the impression—the looks on their faces, the innuendo—that I should be focusing on my family and ought not to be working (paid work, that is).

"But then, you know," Alice continues, "many of the greats have been on their own and just done their own thing; they haven't copied someone else's work. Like I said, here, I try not to see anyone else's work, and I don't show mine, not here."

"I am honoured that you showed me the one you're working on."

"To be honest, you're a writer, not a painter, so it was OK!"

We talk about the range of senses available to perception and memory: sound, for musicians such as her son and Meyer, the painter's sense of the visual, a kinaesthetic sense that Callum and so many others mentioned.

"So the senses sometimes become a part of a picture, are part of the impression. Does it work that way when you read?"

"I think so. I read a great deal when I was growing up. I skimmed a lot; that was my best way of forming a picture."

"You form a picture when you read as well? Like doing a painting, you pick out the details that are important to the general impression."

"Yes, I think that's it, I really do. I mean, now that we're talking about it, I hadn't thought about it before. This is so interesting, things coming together like that. But, you know, I had mentors there too, friends who helped me choose what to read, which was very useful. I never took home any book that wouldn't be useful to me later in school."

"It had to have some sort of relevance or meaning to you right then."

"Yes. It does. Otherwise I wouldn't pay attention."

Conserving Energy

I ask Alice if she has particular ways of remembering everyday kinds of things, such as shopping lists, and she answers that she must "regiment" herself to make sure she locks the doors. Her apartment in Greenwich Village is no longer safe, and she must guard against complacency about what she can do now. On the island she can relax and enjoy herself every minute. "But I think there is a certain amount of fear that comes with living alone in the city, and up here I'm concerned about the roads; the gravel can be treacherous. I face it by being very cautious."

She's concerned about falling; an injury to her leg has meant that she has a tendency to fall back when she gets up from a chair. "I have to do this *[leans forward]* and straighten up as best I can before I start to walk. Otherwise I do this *[bends backwards]*, and I can fall back down a hill. Hard. That's what I did when I cracked my head, and it's the reason everyone's concerned about me and saying, 'Alice, be careful.' And I will. I'm definitely careful."

"So there are these sorts of physical things. Martha has told me that she has had several bad falls because she loses her balance just the way you do. She has an inner ear problem, and that's stressful. I mean you worry, and you're tired for a while afterwards. What about you, are you aware of having less energy?"

"Well, it's a little bit harder to move as quickly. See, I've always done things rather fast and accomplished this and accomplished that and gotten it finished so that I can get to what I want to do."

"Oh, Alice, that sounds so familiar. Get all the housework done so I could read while the children were napping, when I was younger, and now so that I can write, or paint." *I am aware, because of my own situation, of how domesticity and childcare come first for her in the doing and the telling, but her valuing is about her "real work" of painting, as mine is about my writing.*

"Except," I said, "I'm not so good at resting, at letting myself know when I need to rest."

"Oh, well, it will come to you; you'll just fall asleep when you have to *[laughing]*."

Alice tells me she's not accomplishing as much this year as she did last year, when she stayed for the same number of days and did about three paintings a day, more than she has this time. But she is so glad to be here that everything is exciting. The island acts like a "gateway" for her, like Stonehenge did when she saw it, an opening to the spiritual. "Have you ever seen it?" she asks.

"Yes, I have. I was lucky; I was there before they roped it off, and you could go right in and get a sense of the specialness of the place, the spirituality. It sounds to me as if you have always experienced life intensely—more so as you've become older?"

"Well, the only time I've had any problems is when I had to have a hysterectomy, an appendectomy, and a couple of breast operations, that was all."

"All! That sounds like an awful lot."

"Hmmm." She shrugs, in an "Oh, it's nothing" kind of gesture, and nods her head. "I guess so, but you get past those things, don't you. You have to. I think as you grow older, you look more for beauty in ... I hope you do. That would be my hope for most people."

"It sounds as if things are still very fresh for you."

"Well, maybe in an artist's way they are. The rest are the same."

With everyday chores, doing what she has to do, Alice must now be more selective. Since she doesn't accomplish quite as much in a day, she needs to know what she really wants to do. And "stick with that." And she tries to be with younger people, who have more fun and help her "keep up" with the more outgoing side of her life, which is harder to do as you get older. She thinks that's why grandparents and grandchildren are usually so close, because "there's tremendous fun. Do you have grandchildren?" she asks.

"I do. I love being a grandmother—as you say, playing again, and mine certainly keep me on my toes. Their interests open up new interests for me."

"I don't have any yet, but my son is only 40, so I'm still hoping." She goes on to tell me about the three young men who came out on the same boat with her on Sunday and left on Tuesday before she knew they were going to go. When she went for her mail, there was a card from them saying that, besides the seals and the sunset, they had found a new delight. "They meant me!"

"Wonderful!"

"I thought it *was* wonderful. They were from Washington, were here for something, I'm not sure what. You see details like that, when people tell me I might not get them. One was taking pictures all around the island, weather details and the types of characters who were on the island, what is being done on the island and so forth; one was a writer; and the third one—I forget for the moment, but they were three brothers all here for the same thing. And they were so interesting, the things they'd do and say. It stimulates your mind when you're older, because you don't want to let yourself bog down."

"What happens if you do get bogged down?"

"Your spiritual being, your aliveness, your creativeness gets bogged down."

"In what—where are you stuck?"

"You begin to think of your dear ones that have gone. You do, you can't help it, they come back to you; they're very close to you always. I've lost everyone I've ever loved except my darling son and his wife, and my niece, my brother's daughter, in Boston, who helped me get up here. Of course the younger people, thank God, they're there, they're so sweet. I seem to find it very hard to grow old, the fact that you lose so many in death."

Memories of Loss

"It gets lonely, doesn't it?"

"Oh, yes, but you have to avoid that."

"How do you do that?"

"Well, by keeping busy. I really manage pretty well. I have to take care of my own affairs, except that I have somebody who goes over them, the final part of it. I find the fine print, especially in relation to health care, hard to read."

"It *is* hard to read. I find it hard, too. It seems as if they write those directions and then shrink them down to the smallest possible font without reading it themselves. You're 89, and you don't wear glasses?"

"Just for that kind of thing, not for painting."

I ask her whether there are things she remembers now that she didn't before, and she reminisces about the time her brother and sister died. She was sent to an aunt in New York and was away from home for three months. She remembers the horse-drawn trolley and things about New York—such as their first car and the big goggles they wore that didn't prevent all the dust from getting in your face because the cars were open and the roads were mostly dirt.

She pauses for a little while. "I remember how lonely it was. Three months, that was a long time for a little girl. But I didn't talk about that."

"You never mentioned it?"

"No. Everyone was being so kind, and I didn't know— I hadn't quite taken in about my brother and sister. And I missed my mother and father."

"Didn't really realize what had happened, maybe?"

"No, and people didn't want to dwell on it. I guess they thought it would make it worse for me, but I don't know whether it would have."

"Do you remember those feelings, as well as the scenes, in pictures?"

"Oh, yes, how people were around—but not really *there*, you know. Very clear pictures. Always, as far back as I can remember, in pictures. I remember the places I went to be by myself."

Alice tells me that she doesn't recall the past more now than when she was younger unless someone asks her to recall it, like two young women from the art club that want to interview her about Greenwich Village, or "just as we're talking, like now." She doesn't think she's changed mentally. It's that when she's on the island he tends to overdo it, rising early and working hard, and then she'll fall asleep in her chair. "I think that's perfectly normal, don't you?"

"If I got up at 5:30 in the morning, I'd fall asleep in the afternoon for sure. In fact, up here I often have an afternoon nap."

"I never do at home. But dear, up here I get fresh air and not having to go out and buy food and having to carry it home and then cook meals. I'm having a glorious time, in spite of meals at the same time every day."

"Mmmm. Nothing more delicious than other people's cooking."

"And especially dessert. I don't eat dessert at home, but I'm having a little luxury time here. It's silly, isn't it?"

"Why? Everyone deserves a treat now and again. I think it's fun."

"Well," she said, "that's one of the most important things about growing old, is keeping your sense of humour." She thinks that people who get bogged down in all the negatives about growing old (and there are plenty of them) are out of touch with young people and have lost their sense of perspective. She has loads of young friends, especially from the art club. She was the first woman officer in 1923; her club always took in men and women, "so they've always been a broad-minded group, and I've had as much praise from the men as the women."

"It seems to me that your painting is—it's far more than an abiding interest, isn't it?"

"It's a lifetime, just like any composer."

The only time she'd stopped painting was when her husband died. She had turned over the studio to him because he needed a bigger space for some large canvases he was painting. It was very hard for Alice to go back to that studio to work after that. Much later she went back and painted there. "But I never really liked working there. It was too difficult."

"Too many memories?"

"Well, many memories of the person you loved not being there."

"Memories. And feelings of loss. Such a different kind of quiet."

"Oh, yes. And then you remember others—like when my younger sister died. I had expected to go before she did. But I went to my place at Lake George, to the woods and painted, and that was difficult, and so I say to myself ... I mean, loss and sorrow gives more depth maybe in one's work."

"Sometimes you need those breaks where you have to take time off to mourn. This island is one of my places. And Manitoulin Island at home."

"Is it? You do need a place, I know. I have so many memories. But I never stopped painting since then, and I don't plan to, ever. I'll never retire." Like Emma, Alice thinks that people are stupid to retire if they have something they enjoy doing. "People with so many interests can just go on to a new field, a new venture, because, my dear, at 65, you're young! And you're *very* young." *Laughs.* "If only we knew at 65 you aren't old at all ..." *[And now that I'm 83, I see how young I was at 65— how naïve, really]*... "And they're silly if they give up, if they stop doing something, because I think boredom is a killer. See, I'm never bored, ever. I just hope I'm never going to get stuck—it can happen, you know, can take you unawares, like when I come up here, my memories of Bruce are here."

She misses their shared interests and companionship, having someone in your life you know so well, that you don't even have to talk. I tell her that when Martha and I met years ago in one of Claudia's classes, we became good friends almost right away, and how special it is for me to be in touch in the same way. *And now that she's gone, and Miriam and Meyer, and Lev and Russell as well, I am still working up the courage to go back to the island.*

"It is special," Alice agrees, "and it doesn't happen that often. So I think it's a matter of keeping your mind up to a degree of interest."

"And openness?"

"And openness, yes. I find that so many people are so biased, especially in religion. They're hard to talk to."

"And some of them think that getting old is bad. Why do you think that is? Do you think that?"

"That's because they haven't had either the background education or family life that has been … that I had. All the older people in my family were so wonderful."

"Like my mother's friend Beatrice. We have had good models."

"Good models, that's it. I think if a child has had nothing but abuse or difficulties in life, how can they ever have a feeling of love for home or family or the proper relationships that are very important as you grow old?" She doesn't talk with her friends about what it's like to grow old, because they are so much younger and not really interested. But if someone were to ask her, she'd tell them to pick out the things they want to remember about their lives. "Just do the things you like whenever you can. Yourself, nobody else's liking. If it's music, pick out music you like, if it's books, pick out books you like."

I ask her how she would tell people to go about remembering and she says that she remembers herself in her own way and doesn't think you can tell anybody how to remember, exactly.

I agreed that the way each person remembers is unique to them but that she can probably give examples from her life that might trigger someone's memory about theirs. "Like the way you say, 'I just remember in pictures.'"

"Well, I think that's the best way for most people. I think. But then my daughter-in-law has a word memory. She can spell any word. She can write wonderfully."

"Lev remembers somewhat the same way you do, in pictures. Then there's Miriam: she remembers emotions, how she's felt about people. And Meyer remembers the form and character and personality of sounds."

"That's something I would like to be able to do, because I love music. We've talked about opera, and about my sister—who is gone now."

"Yes, we have." The second-sitting diners are wandering into the lounge, and I realize that we've been talking for almost two hours, worry that it's becoming too much for her, and ask her if she is tiring. No, she isn't at all, and if she was she'd let me know! Besides, "This is sort of fun, because I've never really thought about it before this. I haven't thought about myself at all. All my life, I've thought about myself in relation to other people, how they're coming along, especially my son and my daughter-in-law."

"You think about other people, you don't give much thought to yourself ... more to relationships."

"That's right. Except the one time when I was asked to give that talk at my solo show. You see, the older you are, the more important people are. I have some very good friends at the National Arts Club, and they're young, you know. That's where I met the two women—one of them is head of an art centre—who want to write a story about me, and it would be interesting to do that, to talk to them."

I am reminded of Martha as we walked the trails, of Meyer and our conversations by coal-oil lamp, Miriam over lobster rolls at lunch, and all the older people I've talked with, so willing, even eager, to talk about their lives. To tell me their stories. I've done the same really, in my poetry, sculptures, and memoir. Living alone, I welcome the opportunity to talk about my day, in the now and in the past, as Grandma Moses said.

"They feel that I have covered all three wars," Alice continues, "including as a child the Spanish-American, and of course we've had the Korean."

"And the First and Second World Wars."

"The First World War was the most devastating, at least to me, because I lost … I had a friend who was a Canadian ace pilot, and he was killed. I think he was kind of keen about me, and I certainly admired him … I hadn't thought about that for a long time … I think I've told you everything I can think of."

"You've been so generous, told me so much, and given up a whole evening. I know how precious your time is up here, and I'm very grateful."

"Oh, well, it isn't that. I was curious because of the gals wanting to do the story. They found my talk—at the exhibition, you know—interesting. Now I'm much better prepared! I think you've been very nice about it, because you don't make it tiring, you know. You just seem to … just the way in which you ask questions made it possible … I haven't ever had the ability to do this sort of thing."

"What ability is that?"

"Well, discerning …"

"Discerning?"

"Well … making it seem prized, which makes a difference, you see."

Oh Alice, it is you who are the prize in the ways your paintings tell it all, just as you said a good painting does.

One Of

An artist my whole life I came into my own
when I was finally *on* my own, strangely
thriving in the spaces opened
by the deaths that befall the old.

No longer hemmed inside the rules, I paint
commonplace images in a range of methods
and moods;
daring bold colours, translucent for those who
can see
across the fine lines remaining.

It's what we do, we women, we express
the nitty-gritty of everyday life, until it is
allowed—
we are obliged to find a way—to bleed across
loss
running the gamut of all that matters, held
matted together.

An old, old woman I go out at dawn into the
woods
or wait by the sea, the colour saturated until
rendered down
to exactly the beauty *I* want seen
yielding to the canvas, painted

in the snatched moments of quiet in my studio.
It's what we do.

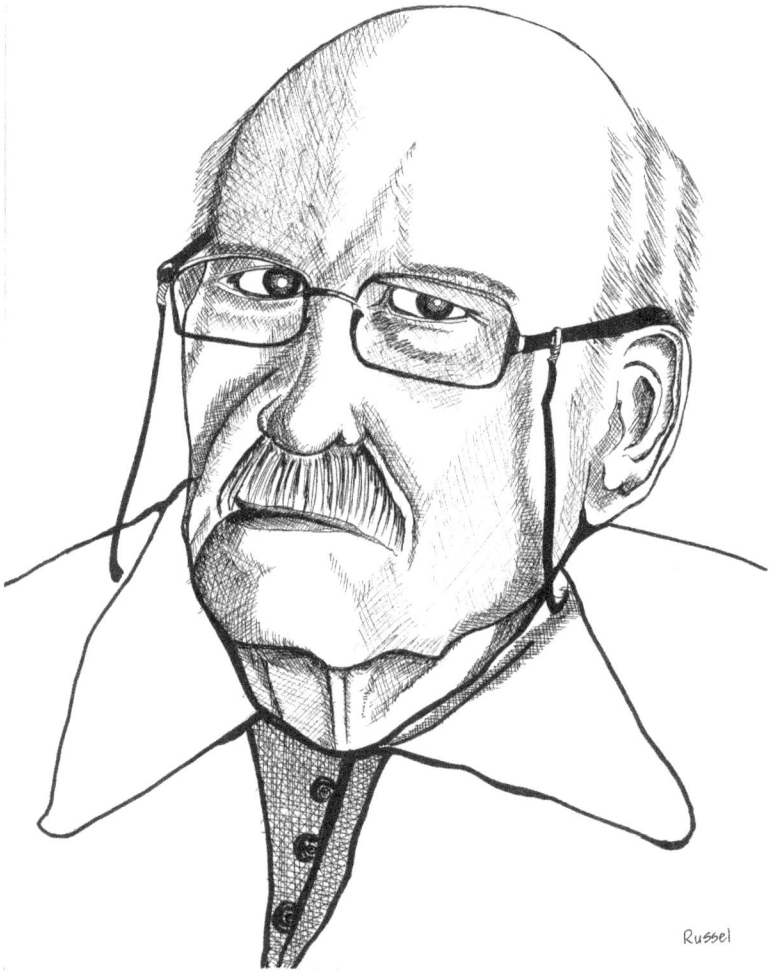

Russel

Another Back-Door Entrance: Russell's Story

"The one big tragedy of my childhood, the tragedy of my life, is being dyslexic. I cannot think in the usual way."

Seagulls swoop down from the rookery high
on the island's rocky back-side,
white-grey in cloud or sun they circle the laden ferry
squawking for food as she nears the dock.
Woods, meadow, and gardens fenced
from deer are green. Fisher houses,
weathered grey and old,
are tucked on the inward curve from school house to
church,
white to white, points of definition,
like folded wings.
Houses of summer people climb hills. They live more on
rock,
higher, in sight of water and distance and their other
lives.
On the low side

one road, barely two miles long, from harbour
to farthest cove. Too rough for bicycles,
fit for stout shoes and bare feet curling, or a golf cart
for those who can no longer negotiate the surface
or walk its two-mile length.

Whatever the Mind Creates

Everybody says there are more summer people on the island than there used to be, but, according to Russell, "It's whatever your mind creates—Oh, one or two more houses every three or four years. In the same way there are only so many beds, and you have to sleep on a bed or you get fined $60. There's no camping allowed because of the risk of fire. The two boats can carry just so many, and you can't get any more people on the island. We're self-limited. When people say there are a lot more—houses, people, and so forth—they have just become conscious of them, I think."

Some days he feels crowded by "people with giant cameras or boy scouts who come for a day" invading a favourite place. Waiting for the return boat, they picnic on the grass in front of the inn, "with the owner glaring at them. But they won't be there tomorrow."

Russell's house is the only one on the island not muted to grey by wind and sea-salt. Bright pink, it stands against rock, an exclamation, visible in all weather. Laundry flaps above on a drying rack anchored in a small patch of grass in the rocks. Chairs and a table wait under a folded sun-umbrella. One day, after a not-too-tiring or -sweaty hike, I notice a sign beside the door: "Felice House, 2:00—4:30 Weekdays Only," and decide to stop by.

Bells on the screen door jangle as I step down into the small, bright kitchen crammed with a neatly arranged clutter of crockery and utensils—for Russell's home, "too much is not enough." Around the end of a counter, past a beaded curtain on the left, I step up over a high doorsill into the studio where he sits stitching at a large table by the window. Behind him, layered skeins of wool hang in rainbow colours, ranging from deep purple to pale red. In the corner, music plays. In front and to his right on walls and tables, Mexican jewellery and cloth from winter sojourns, now for sale.

He gives me a quick look, eyes bright blue and huge through the thick glasses required by encroaching glaucoma, his hair a white tonsure above a narrow and ascetic face accented with a short, grey bristle of moustache. He continues to work, using a magnifying glass for one eye, a bright light over the canvas.

Needle and wool shape forms of ancient Aztec, Mayan, and Toltec glyphs traced on the canvas from his "in-situ drawings." His fingers work rhythmically in a random stitch he invented on the island and calls Libra Point, "because it's foolproof, anyone can do it. When I went to classes I couldn't remember what they taught me, it's impossible for me to follow a set pattern. So I had to invent a way to do it and made up my own stitch. You can't tell from the front that it's different from the usual way, but you can from the back, because it's a mess. If you pull it apart, you find that it's based on a whole structure of error: that it looks okay is some kind of mystery, and a form of compensation."

I come to know him through watching him stitch. He explains that he can teach Libra Point to "ultra-handicapped people" because the stitch "is random, spontaneous, and yet risk-taking—it's different." Through our conversations I begin to see how learning and teaching this unique kind of stitchery are like a memory thread of his life.

A Life of Struggle
A Constant Challenge

Both of Russell's parents were from well-known Philadelphia merchant families, Quaker for several generations, but descended from Scotch Covenanters who had emigrated in the 17th century because their faith was too extreme to fit with the Jacobean compromises of the time. Russell and I used the same words to describe our heritage, echoing each other:

"Dreadful Scotch Presbyterian, with all the WASP consciousness and conscience."

"The Puritan work ethic," I reply. "To produce is the only way to …"

"Yes, we have to, until our dying day."

"You still feel that way?" I ask.

"Of course, don't you?"

"Well, I fight it—I try to find things to be task-oriented about that are a bit pleasanter for me."

"No point in fighting it," Russell says. "What's the matter with pessimism?"

The point of his stitching needle recalls for him his five-year-old bitten fingernail tracing an X, and then he tells me how his dyslexia first manifested itself: "I had a job reading. The first word I think I ever knew, when I was about five years old, was Mexico. I had a jug my missionary uncle had sent to our family, and in the middle of a word on the jug was the letter X, and I would go over it with my bitten fingernail across the X. Why I had that compulsion I haven't the faintest idea; it was a sensory thing I suppose, of some kind. And then, so, I kind of got to be conscious of the other letters around it, and when I was with my two favourite cousins, whom I hardly knew, but whom I liked very much, I got to know the word Mexico. That time was buried in the unconscious for all these years until this winter, when I was writing an article, and all of a sudden I realized my early connection with Mexico."

This memory pulled other memories of photographs sent back to Philadelphia by the same family, of the names of places where they lived and where some of the people in his life now dwelled. "It made a very nice picture … a nice paragraph in the article I was writing. Now that I'm writing, it's all coming back to me, and I'd rather it didn't. I've put those years behind me, and they're not welcome."

No one dared tell his mother or his aunt, both of them teachers, that although he seemed right he had "lots of disability." And he didn't dare, because he knew he'd get into trouble with his father, so he hid in the classroom, enough to be forgotten, not catch the teacher's eye, and for a while he just slipped through. "What happened," he tells me, "was I *heard* my education." His grandfather liked to read aloud, and Russell *wanted* to read, so he "exploited" him, by listening to him and learning to read through sound, from the intonation and rhythm of his voice. He was about 13 when his grandfather stopped reading aloud, so he had to do it himself. "I could grasp the beginning and end of a word, but not the middle … I learned to get that by inference. But when I tried to *say* the words out loud, they were unrecognizable. So of course I was found out. My father and grandfather thought I was stupid and lazy, and the teachers thought I was subnormal.

"But *I* always had a pretty good sense of my own intelligence, even though I never passed an exam. And when my mother and my aunt, both teachers, finally recognized that, they believed in it and persuaded the teachers that I belonged in school. They got me in again by the back door, and I got around the exams. Otherwise they wouldn't have kept me."

He didn't want to be *different*, didn't *want* anyone to think he was lazy or stupid, so he practised until it came out without too much hesitancy. But when it came to taking in something new, he was in trouble. He had to make things up to sound like the original, which worked only in spontaneous situations. But not well enough to get by in school. He still loses words when he reads aloud.

The kind of abstract thinking that requires an answer to a question or an organized, thoughtful comment—*that* involved being able to follow a logical train of thought. And that's not the way he thinks.

(*I notice that when I ask him a question, especially one involving feelings, he'll say, "I don't know," or "I couldn't care less," and then a few minutes later give an opinion or an answer in a colourful, kinaesthetic description of the person or event.*)

Reading was difficult for him, but writing was worse; it bordered on a foreign language. He couldn't remember lots of words, and so he'd use a synonym, and it came out cumbersome and convoluted, with the end of the sentence often coming before the beginning ... like German. "Oh, well," he laughs, "if you have enough mumbo-jumbo, people don't know what you're talking about anyway." He thinks that Gertrude Stein and James Joyce probably had some sort of handicap, because they would write in such a convoluted way only to answer a need of theirs to compensate. "They're unreadable because we don't recognize their symbols.

"So, you see, dyslexia is not so hidden, it's obvious to others when you can't perform verbally, which is what people set store on. Numbers are always a problem. I can't make change—just have to rely on people's being honest. But it doesn't take the whole person over completely. You learn to go past, through, and around the incomprehensible. You learn to compensate."

"Sounds creative, like Libra Point."

"Nonsense. What's creative about it? I can tell when other people are doing it. Clever maybe, but not creative."

As happened with his memory of X and Mexico, writing brought back memories for him—often the bitter ones of his childhood. He doesn't think being an only child made much difference, that he would have been jealous if there had been siblings, who might have been "normal." He just took it because he was a child.

There was so much he didn't understand. At first that he was *not*—not like others, not as smart, not as hard-working. And then he was bewildered about why he didn't have understanding teachers or therapists who could *name* his problem and who could help him with it, even overcome it. He couldn't pass into the senior year of high school, but they graduated him anyway, probably because they didn't know what else to do with him, he says.

Finding His Way

He took himself to New York, to theatres and art shows, but he "lost face," felt he was a social outcast, and always has been. "If the problem had been faced in childhood … but it was hidden … ignored … made fun of. I did not have the support I needed … *surely* some teacher could have been found to help me overcome my disability … to find a place."

His vocational test in high school showed a talent for education and religion, and he went to theological college and succeeded because there weren't too many tests. Poor writing skills barred him from teaching, and he worked in settlement houses with children, and then as director of education at a small religious school. Bored, he went to art school. He wasn't good at drawing, "which is more like words," but he was good at design and watercolour. Watercolour wasn't considered real art then, but the genre "obsessed" him for a while and proved useful in his work with children, and later with disturbed adolescents, which he did for 29 years. He had the opportunity to work with a well-known children's art therapist in New York, and became the first psychoanalytically oriented children's art therapist in the city. He liked working with groups, not classes, "where people could find a place and work freely."

He tells me about a lecture he gave, and discovering that the more he talked the more easily he spoke, and the less he talked the more hesitancy there was. "The channels weren't there for me, I had to clear out the channels—depends on the audience, some chemical business in the atmosphere. My wall hangings were the limbs on which I hung my talk and some days the talk would be completely different. I'd be surprised the way the children responded; they would surge towards me like a wave, some of them hardly walking, but keeping up, and would kiss me, circling around me saying: 'Gracias, gracias.' That was a rewarding, sensitive experience for me. Art therapy was another obsession, if you like … you live it, and that's part of your life, you're not satisfied unless you're doing it. It was my kind of therapy because there's no need to interpret, to verbalize or externalize the picture. In sensing it, you experience it—the drawing or the art product itself is a form of language, and many times that's all that's necessary. Most therapists dig (ask questions) because they're verbal. But you don't have to do that, just be willing to wait. In painting, the mind is not trained to censure visual material because it's entirely its own language. I had to train myself not to see symbolic meanings, which are really my meanings, not theirs."

Russell and Callum would have agreed with each other about having no difficulty remembering art and music that was "felt through" and that communicating in a visual or auditory way (such as music) is language.

"How did you do that, not intrude yourself?"

"You just make it up as you go along, based on who the person is. When you see an aesthetic problem in the painting, you use that as a way to reach them. The verbal is useful only for him to bring what he's painted to another level, so he can see what he's saying in the painting ... catharsis ... then you'll get to another layer, you hope. You get layer on layer. I can always spot a dyslexic in their artwork."

"How?"

"They're unconventional, or they try to be conventional and can't, because they don't use the usual patterns. You can see it.

"I gave up watercolour after a while. Now I'm retired from therapy. The stock answer is that I didn't have time, that I had no more patience with it. The real answer is that I'm committed to whatever I'm doing now. Stitching took the place of watercolour. I'm just wondering what happens when I go blind."

A Life in Stitches

Russell recalls that when he first saw Mexican glyphs the "design and colour punched me in the face," but when I refer to this response in another conversation he barks, "Those aren't my words."

I had asked him if I could tape our conversations, to help me remember. He thought it was a great idea and wished he'd "had that technology 50 years ago." Now I ask if I can refer back to the tape. His curiosity overcomes his reluctance, I find the particular section on the tape and play it back: "Well, it's hard to believe I said that. I don't say things like that. Glyphs are dynamic forms that are easily seen, easily worked by people who have no sense of design, no so-called artistic sense, if there is such a thing. The dramatic transfer to canvas from the standpoint of colour relationships made me shiver."

"An emotional ... a physical response to ...?" I begin.

"It's an immediate reaction to the *space* to be used, but that's not creative—the image isn't coming from inside. I'm using existing space, rearranging, recomposing the material in my own way so it's like making comments, rather than being original, although it's not a copy."

He also sharply denies the connection he had made in our earlier conversation between his finger tracing the X on the Mexican jug as a child, his adult love of Mexico and the glyphs, and the similarity he discovered between stitches and words when he took up needlepoint, how stitches are a language of their own: "That's crap, a fabrication, too appropriate, bordering on the sentimental and gushy. Junk. What people like to read. You create fiction from your own experience by embroidering it a little bit."

"And yet you say a painting has its own language."

"That's different, that would be original."

"Surely the glyphs were original in their own time."

"Well, yes." Laughs. "You've got me! While it's mainly pictorial, there is a linguistic aspect in it, there are word signs which you have to look up in the dictionary, which I can't do, so I just work at realizing what they are and then begin to put them together, like detective work. Each glyph has its own language. Now C. [one of his students] made me really angry, she was altering the design, and so she was distorting the language."

"And who knows what it says when you do that?"

"Yes. She's more dyslexic in colour than I am in English. I told her I'd tear up her work and do it myself if she did it again. I wouldn't want anyone to speak bad English to me. I'd rather they speak in their own language and let me guess at what they're saying."

"As you've done all your life—and do with the glyphs."

"I suppose. People put too much value on words anyway. The only original thing I do now is decide how I treat someone else's material. It's not creative, it's just filling in."

"But they are *your* designs—*your* response to the space, your way of seeing the relationships—your choice of how you will make that dramatic transfer of colour to canvas."

"I didn't think of it first."

"Libra Point is original!"
"Well, yes, but it's a compensation."
"You seem to enjoy it though."
"You mean satisfaction."
Good old Puritan!

An Island and Mexico

Russell first went to the island to paint—"with a weird entourage, a one-eyed worker with a licence who couldn't drive, and a 13-year-old schizophrenic who could, but was not supposed to." He was on sabbatical, looking for something more stimulating than teaching, and there they were on a speck of an island, "coming back to earth, to the middle of nowhere, a hole in the woods. I gave myself a place to work as freely as all those disadvantaged kids I taught. The price of my sabbatical was to write a monograph on my methods of teaching them."

With "enormous self-discipline," he "painted and wrote, wrote and painted." The monograph was officially rejected because group art therapy was not thought possible at the time. Subsequently the material was used throughout the children's mental health system as a teaching model. Someone else published his material and mentioned him in the bibliography, "which is really all that matters, because the authors' names are forgotten and the reference is not. Once your name is there, you're safe. But I would have liked the pleasure of giving the paper."

During his middle years, as he added weeks to each visit, his fantasy of being rich enough to spend the entire summer on the island expanded to include dreams of winters in Mexico. At first he had to have an excuse (*Puritans have a hard time with holidays and leisure*). His was that he wanted to see the place where the designs came from. Then friends invited him to visit. He didn't really want to stay at Comitán, because of V. "I've been under dominating, castrating women all my life: not my mother especially, although she didn't push hard enough for me, but teachers and bosses who have been pioneer women in the fields of art, the handicapped and education … some unconscious fulfilment … can't dig it up … don't want to. But I ended up very close to V." Last year he was artist in residence, and this year he will have a show there.

Russell retired in 1976, a year that marked his "B.C. and A.D." At first he had gone to the island in "bitter weather," stretching the time between as long as possible. "Now I don't have to punish myself that way any longer and choose to come when it pleases me." He's so busy that he wonders how he ever had time to work. Now that he "knows what to do"—over the years he has learned how to write "publishable material"—he would "like to go back to the crack of a school bell."

When he leaves the island in autumn, he goes first to his home in Philadelphia, where he lives "in between" with Ian, his lifelong companion, near the scene of his early working years as a social worker in settlement houses. Then he goes on to Comitán, drawn there by those "objective designs" that punch him in the face, and by his earliest memories—of family, of learning, of flesh.

Are there sea shells and lobster buoys in the living room at Comitán? As I listen to Russell talk about his life, similar aspects in me surface that I had never before seen so clearly. And I realize how ambiguous our Puritan, patriarchal background is. While it has shaped us, our attitudes, our aspirations, our lives, it has not supported or nurtured us in the achievement of more iconoclastic goals or to feel worthwhile in our choices. It does not hold us up. It is the island that has held us up—as rock-hard and unyielding as our heritage, and a relentlessly inescapable place, where body must be remembered for survival, and from which to grow: a "hole in the woods" wall where we can "come back to earth."

"A Lot of Bunk."
Thinking, Memory, and Aging

As for aging, Russell grumbles, "There's a lot of bunk in what people believe. That whole thing about 'frantic elders' is a stereotype, although there's a grain of truth in it, otherwise it wouldn't be there. The weakest spot goes to the extreme, and so the problems you've always had become more so as you get older—like all the other problems constellated around my dyslexia, emotional and so on, not noticed at the time. If I'd worked at it more, taken better care of myself, maybe it wouldn't have been so bad. But you can't do something about what you don't notice."

Russell thinks that true memory is *about* thinking, and, since he cannot think "in the usual way," he claims to possess a poor memory. He talks about two kinds of memory: "Rote, fuelled by fear of performing and getting a grade, which is gone after the exam, which I can't do anyway," and attention to "quality—pitch, rhythm—which is inferential, related to the sensory, like a musician. I became a very good listener and could pick up on verbal intonation and so forth."

"How is this not thinking in the usual way?"

"It's not thinking. I remember constellations, contexts of events, feelings, and people. This is just trivia about events, not like remembering particulars such as names and dates, or following a logical argument."

He doesn't mention the sensory aspects of memory, although he has practised them all his life. He learned to read through listening, and to write through touch; he taught children by moving with them; used artistic media rather than words in therapy. He invented a Libra Point language understood sensuously like other artistic media. And he remembers through contexts, constellations, and relationships.

He is sure that art, and the sensory, are not only a means of expressing feelings but are also powerful ways of understanding in a different way and communicating in a different kind of language. However, since this way is not "logical"—sequential and factual—it has nothing to do with "real" thinking or memory as he conceives them.

In fact, he considers his way of relational thinking that comes from seeing something in nature, or in a glyph, and making it in a language other people can understand, has little to do with creativity. He doesn't even look at his own inventions as creative because they are a "compensation" for having to find ways around his disability, or because they are more "women's" crafts and skills, like his inspired cooking, his amazing house, even stitchery itself.

Not until his work appeared in group or one-man shows and began to sell could he legitimate it as artwork, as worthwhile, as worth his own and other people's effort. Though not cognitive, nor the kind of real profession and place he wanted in the masculine world, art as a money-maker could enter the world of "real work." We were talking one day about the Puritan notion that money legitimizes human endeavour, and I said, "Now you've joined the clan."

"What do you mean?"

"Well, the family firm."

With a short bark of a laugh he looks at me slyly, "My grandfather would be upright in his grave with outrage to hear you say that. My father would just be disgusted. Another back door entrance, eh?" He laughs again.

Memory Loss

According to Russell, memory loss can occur at any age: "That's obvious—if I don't pay attention to reading a page, I'm not going to remember what I've read; everyone does this, more so when you're old."

"Why? Because you notice it more?"

"I don't know ... but, if I have no use for it, I forget it, like I never remembered dates." His grandfather was a historian, so names and dates were important to him, and he encouraged Russell to remember things. Russell refused to credit them as important and didn't pay attention. His grandfather was careless with him; forgetting names and dates was Russell's way of "hitting him over the head." Now that he has a use for them, dates of shows and so on, they matter to him, and so he tries harder. But he hasn't acquired the habit. He observes that you use it or lose it and that old people forget more because they don't have much to remember. They're not active mentally; they have no interests, spend their time watching TV.

"We're full of ease on memory, and yet at the same time it can be a stumbling block in the simplest way, like losing words. It's probably anxiety, and that makes you feel disconnected." His most frightening experience, then and now, is talking to someone and forgetting completely what he means to say, such as a high school experience he had of going on stage and forgetting everything he'd taken such a long time to memorize. "It was embarrassing … I lost face … everybody thought I was stupid. Anxiety halts the memory process at any age, derails it, is a waste of emotional effort. I don't like the way my memory is to my disadvantage when I do this, because old memories come up and make me lose track of the narrative. I'm remembering more details of my past, just like my grandfather used to do, and I hate it. These people were part of my childhood. And not a very good part."

Any strategies to "get around" memory loss he considers "devious tricks, dishonest, hiding your faults and exploiting other people," like the ones he used to manage his dyslexia. A few things are legitimate aids, such as sleep, which rests his mind, and "supercharged energy exchanges between people, as with friends, or in a massage. There's a wonderful person here on the island. I don't pay any attention to those crystals of hers and all that junk, but I leave feeling better than I've any right to expect. Developing techniques like this to remember is important to a lot of people. If I cared more I'd have a system, my own form of mythology—everybody's system has some sort of rightness.

"And you must take care of yourself—a constant, lonely battle—nobody understands or cares about old people; I don't myself. Of course, we become obsessed with money, what else is there? The young are going to get there, they should be taught to value elders, see their needs. You're thrown on your own. I was from the beginning.

"I have this fantasy about a foundation that gives money to older people, people beyond the pale—which I was as a kid, and now am again from the standpoint of age—to help with the chores that get in the way of my work ... so that they might finish the creative job that they've started and can't continue because of financial circumstances ... somebody ought to have that kind of foundation."

He looks over at me, lost face smiling slightly. I can see that he is tense, even though he says he has "gone over this stuff so much that it doesn't mean anything emotionally" to him anymore. As usual, we look at his day's work and then walk past the kitchen counter, through a door curtained in glass beads, into a living room whose space is lit with the hot colours of Mexico. Mexican designs stitched in wool on covers and cushions, on objets d'art and memorabilia precisely placed on walls and tables, with a practised eye for the most telling effects. Fisherman's Glass and other sun catchers float in every window; on the sills, old green glass bottles in varying shapes and sizes with a fat red tomato perched on top of each one. The walls, like the ones of his childhood, are "held up with books." For me, overwhelming, but for him "too much is never enough." It never was.

We have tea and homemade cookies, and he gives me an article he has written about his Mexican work, "Artist in the House of Jaguars," and tells me that another writer suggested the title should be "WASP in the House of Jaguars." I laugh, and he, mistaking my delight for criticism, barks: "I didn't think that was funny, I thought it was very nice."

"It's marvellous!"

"Because I'm a WASP, I think I have the right to say it."

"You sure do!"

Russell's Contradictions

The longer I knew Russell, the more his kindness and caring for other people cracked through the crust of irascibility and cynicism. He is a patient, and with children, a loving teacher. He has a lifelong partner. He's a gourmet cook, loves to entertain, is a skilled interior designer, and a dedicated gardener. I was often on the receiving end of his thoughtfulness: he knew that I was on my own on the island and over the years unobtrusively made sure I met people, made quiet suggestions about out-of-the-way places to explore that weren't too demanding physically. And he tolerated with good grace my curiosity about his life and his views on art, therapy, and aging, and many other questions. He has many friends and makes memorable contributions in several worlds, and yet, if he thinks about himself in these ways, you would never know it from the way he talks about his life.

For example, by imagining himself to be rich, he "fantasized" the island and Mexico from yearning reverie into places where he now lives. While he can now be in these loved places for as long as he wants to, he "has burnt up the fantasy so I can't get a good one anymore." His designs of glyphs in Libra Point "language" are well-known, exhibited in group and one-man shows, and stitched and taught nationally. Even so, now that he "is an old man, the memories that remain ... are the ashes of childhood" and "the struggles to make something" of himself.

This contradiction between his accomplishments and his attitude about his life and career surfaced early on in our conversations and became increasingly puzzling to me. He is furious when I ask whether learning to read and write in a sensory way might have had a positive, though unforeseen, outcome, by providing him with a kind of childhood training in the sensory as a means of communication and expression. That it may have shaped his kind of artwork and the way he remembers. I am surprised at his vehemence—it's not an unusual question to ask a psychoanalytically oriented therapist. However, he seems to assume that I am inferring that he has not worked through his childhood feelings and glares at me, "I've told the story so many times that all of the feeling has gone out of it ... there's nothing there." But the bitter past does seem to live on in his feelings of there being nothing there and that too much is never enough.

Life was hard for Russell. He was right in his opinion that he didn't fit in to the standard expectations of success for men, that he had to work harder than most to learn, to earn a living, at his art, and to accomplish his dreams. But he *was* supported, and by many people.

His mother and aunts, and later a series of teachers and mentors, recognized his considerable abilities, recognized the way he *did* think, through what he called their "intuition." They opened up opportunities for him, and some sponsor his shows now. He has had many successes: teacher, loved social worker, art therapist, director of well-known educational and art therapy institutes, and recognized stitcher and writer about stitching art. He is reticent about, but proud of, his students' successes, and proud enough to downplay, in that familiar, self-deprecating way, his recent shows in Mexico and the United States. He has invented a popular and saleable art form and been able to realize his dream of living on the island in summer and in Mexico in winter. He has accomplished his dreams through his own gifts, energy, and work. He *does* have a legitimate and acknowledged place.

But he gives scant credit to the women who saw his potential and went to bat for him, or who later bought his house so that he could live rent-free in the summer and still have some money. For Russell, all of this is no substitute for his being able to think cognitively and have a place in that world. They could not forge that entry for him. Their belief in him and their appreciation of his abilities opened up opportunities for him, but in a world he believed to be inferior.

And he has a point. The intellectual world, often thought of as a masculine domain even today, is the most usual realm of recognition, respect, and material success. With as much help as was available at the time, and with a great deal of hard work and persistence, Russell found a place. But it is not the place he wants in the "real" world of work, not the kind of help he wanted, nor the men from whom he wanted it. In spite of praise and success in social service, education, and art, he dwells on the people and system that did not support him.

And he focuses on his frustrations and regrets, not on his satisfaction with what he has accomplished and the persistence and creativity required; on how not being able to "think in the usual way" barred him from the world he so coveted, not on the worlds he has opened for himself. His internal sadness about not having "made something of himself" in the world he longed to be part of overshadows his accomplishments and the support he received along the way. Because in so many ways the world denied to him *was* more important, he was unable to see or appreciate his talents, hard work, and courage.

And so he "does not have good memories of his life." His pervasive perception of himself as inadequate, forged in the social milieu in which teaching children, the social services, and art were not viewed as masculine values or practices, colours his entire life with the greyness of disappointment.

And yet. The contradictions between his perceptions of himself and his long and obviously successful life are so marked, and so often in his own awareness, that I am left with an uneasy feeling of having had the wool pulled over my eyes. Neither Puritan Covenanters nor Quakers are given to self-praise. Could it be that Russell's persistently negative talk about himself does not match his feelings about himself? He remembers having "had a pretty good sense of" his own intelligence. Does he also have a "pretty good" appreciation of his art and his accomplishments but no way, no language or framework, from within which a man could talk about them? He certainly knows that the unconventional artistic ways he did find—which he calls compensatory rather than creative—had little chance of receiving acknowledgment in the "real" (masculine) world of work, at least in his younger days. But no longer. Now his work is well recognized.

On a late August day Russell and Ian depart the island on the morning boat. Everyone is at the dock to say goodbye. There is a tradition for summer residents and visitors leaving the island at the end of their stay. A friend will give them a few flowers— never wild flowers, never picked oneself. As the boat sails around the harbour to make the second turn, which heads her out to sea, they throw the flowers on the water to ensure a return to the island. As people continue to wave, they watch Russell and Ian. No flowers are strewn on the water. They will not be back.

Legacy

There are more than two boats a day travelling
to the island now, and more people than
before.
The trails worn down from too many feet,
the island, dried-out tired by August, shrinks
into itself.

The pink house is still there, still Felice House:
bought years ago by friends as he grew poor,
its ground floor now a store, selling wine,
cheeses,
and fresh produce to a gourmet clientele.
The rent goes towards a foundation

for two young artists to live and work every
year
under the eaves, where Russell and Ian
slept. The row of yellow ducks still peers from
the bathtub's rim when we view their summer's
work.

Canvases stitched in random "foolproof"
Libra Point grew out of this rock-hard island
his Mother Earth freedom home, then Russell
left for Mexico, place
of punching colours and designs to shiver in.

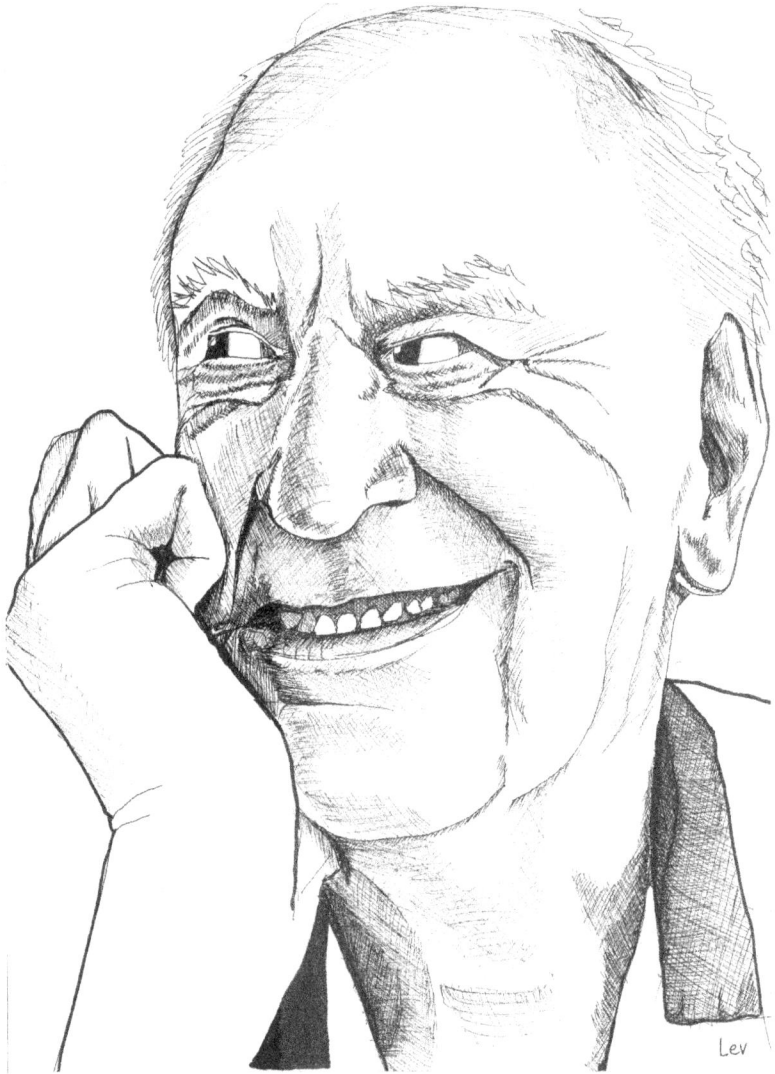

Brush In Hand: Lev's Story

"With every loss there is a gain, and contrariwise."

A Great Raconteur

W alk up the gravel road past the four corners where the church, the post office, the Island Hostel, and the general store meet. The road narrows, the stones are bigger, ready to trip over; wild roses fence in houses on either side. There's a big red-painted house on the left as you turn a corner, and on your right a sign points up a hill to an old hotel, the last building you'll see before the big grey house looking over the ocean and the rusty-ribbed shipwreck keeled over on the rocky shore.

By dinner time Lev can be found in the communal dining room sitting with a group of painters, laughing and talking after their day's work. My first day there he waved me over, introduced me all around, asked me where I was from, why I was visiting, and teased me about being one of the "breathers," the nickname for students in sensory awareness classes.

For three precious weeks, Lev stays in a weathered white clapboard cottage with a green peaked roof down a grassed hill from the main building, closer to the coast road and the sounds and smells of the sea—black-backed gulls wheeling and crying overhead announce the fishing boats he loves to paint coming into harbour. Because of a serious heart condition, Lev stays in the only ground-floor room, with access to the staff toilet and laundry. Every evening, painters gather around the fireplace in the parlour across from his room to critique each other's work. Bystanders, which I often am, are welcome to listen. Lev is always in the thick of it, a stocky, muscular man, white-haired, with tan lines wrinkling around his gleaming brown eyes as he laughs or makes a point. Loving every minute.

Being with interesting people and getting out—into nature and away from meager surroundings—have always been critical for Lev. To escape New York City summers he went on camping trips with his parents, and later with his son. His heart condition rules out camping now, and even much walking, and so the island—nature, spirit, creativity, and companionship—are his only way out and "talking and arguing with the people here" his "breath of life."

He is an entertaining raconteur himself, and I often join him and his friends as they hash over everything from philosophy, politics, and painting techniques to island goings on. Lev is a storehouse of information and argues his point of view knowledgeably, decisively, and with great conviction, but never defensively—always eager to learn. He never loses the thread of his argument, and neither do we, because he enlivens it with anecdotes in vivid word pictures that are always "right to the point."

He came late to painting and taught himself, except for weekly life-drawing lessons at New York's Museum of Modern Art that painter friends from the island told him about, reassuring him that anyone could attend—seniors for free. When the subway's escalators broke down and he couldn't use the stairs because of his "wonky heart," his friends drove him to class, and they would all have lunch afterwards to talk about the day's work. The techniques he learned were an eye opener, and learning something new at every class was exciting. Even better were the creative people he met, "wise no matter what their age; the way they look at things, like seeing the spaces between things as full of energy, that there was no such thing as empty air! And artists are more likely to go out on a limb, experiment. Well, about some things, anyway," he laughs. "Artists have their dogmas, too."

Whenever we talk, usually sitting on the front porch waiting for dinner, or afterwards, walking down to the cove to watch the sunset, Lev regales me with stories about his life. I listen, fascinated by his stories, and by the *way* they come to his mind: "I might not remember a book right after I've read it, but when I hear a key word, in a flash I see it all; without a key word or incident, if I stand on my head, I can't remember it." Like many of the older people I talked to, what is memorable for Lev is a new or vivid event or an insight into people: "Then I can tell the story. It's like recalling a key argument and putting it together with my own point of view." I am enthralled by the way he follows his theme (or the essence, as he calls it) through a maze of details and sidetracks, keeping associations appropriate to his focus and discarding the rest, "leaving his brain free" for what is important to the story he is telling.

When I comment that he paints pictures with his words, Lev looks puzzled, saying that he remembers what helps him understand the way people think or act the way they do, recalls memories of past events, or what he read, on the thread of his own interest in them. "This is an entirely verbal process, there's nothing pictorial there for me at all." But in his descriptions of *how* he remembers, the verbal, pictorial, and kinaesthetic meet: "All right, as I'm talking to you now, I see the chairman at work, the union chairman. I see this other individual, they're talking about him, they're laughing, he's laughing. I see the whole thing, and then these people come over to me—it's all there, like a film unrolling, as if it were from a script for TV. And that's the way I see most of these things."

A Tough Life

Lev's parents were Russian Jewish immigrants, "the only Christ killers in a WASP town"—a small place with an iron foundry. He was bullied and beaten at school and ostracized in the neighbourhood. Every Sunday the family "got out of town," going on long walks in the country to escape the noise and filth of the iron foundry that "infected the air" and the uneasiness of constantly feeling different and isolated. Lev tells me that his father was tough, a European-trained tailor, with years of rugged apprenticeship: non-conformist, anti-establishment, and anti-religious—perhaps the ground of Lev's atheism, so vividly reinforced by a terrible scene from his childhood.

When he was nine years old, he saw a group of Protestant men set fire to the nativity scene in front of a Roman Catholic church. He could "see those men chopping up the fire hoses, the water spurting out and making frozen puddles on the ground, so none of the nativity scene could be saved." He tells me he expected God to throw a thunderbolt on the town, and he'd see it destroyed. When it wasn't, he wondered, "What's the matter with God that he doesn't take care of his property? This is the root of my atheism. I am a Jewish atheist who believes in the teachings of Jesus Christ."

They moved to New York to find better-paid jobs for both parents. In good times, they lived with his father's customers while he made entire wardrobes for the whole household—a week in the spring and a week in the autumn for each home. His mother usually cooked for the family and during the lean summer and winter her cleaning and cooking jobs often provided their only income.

"She was different," Lev tells me, "very European, the way she spoke, in her dress, her cooking—that's why they loved her for their parties. And she was adventurous, she listened to opera, and she loved to sing: I remember the lullabies she sang to me when I was little, and I love opera to this day, the sound of those voices gives me the shivers. But she worked like a damned drudge all her life. No matter how hard she tried, there was never enough." And so Lev grew up knowing both worlds, the rich and the poor, especially the poor. All his life, he "felt like an odd ball, on the fringe. I wore the clothes my father made, I had to, we could never afford to buy clothes, but they were too good for Harlem. I was ashamed to go out in the street."

Lev's father had very demanding standards—he was "stubborn, and he always had a good opinion of himself. Although no one appreciated it, *he* knew he was a better tailor than anyone trained in New York. Maybe that's why he was hard to get along with, always had to be right." Lev says he felt that he himself never measured up, was always expected to do better, at school and later at work. His father "was never physical, but we fought a lot when I got older. But you know," he laughs, "it was good training; at least I learned not to take anything for granted!"

Lev left school at 16 to help support his family and apprenticed at the *New York Times* with one of his father's friends. He loved getting to know the writers he admired, thought of their discussions as a continuation of his education, and stayed with the *Times* all his working life, eschewing any promotion that would cut him off from this camaraderie. Admired for his prodigious memory—his colleagues called him a memory machine—and for his interests in the arts, he felt part of a professional group, if only "on the fringe." "Leaving school at 16 'wasn't a big deal,'" says Lev—"everyone else was doing it"; but he wanted to continue his education and one of his teachers suggested that he read philosophy and the classics. He and two friends met every week to discuss Hegel, Marx, Spinoza, and some of the great poets, such as Wordsworth. They "groaned about the tough reading" at first, but persevered: he was learning how to think, how to figure things out, "how to remember to get the essence, the juice, out of something that's important. Instead of trying to remember everything, I just tried to remember that which had some meaning for me."

Lev went to the public library at least twice a week; the librarians came to know him and recommended books. He remembers one volume in particular, a life of Isadora Duncan. He called her "Mother Courage" because her story gave him the courage to deal with his problems and to go to concerts and ballet—"not a guy thing with my friends," he laughs. Much later, he wrote to me: "I have just seen a broadcast of The Kirov Ballet. It was almost unbelievable to watch the lead move like a bit of poetry, like a melody. My inside was just welling up with emotion, watching the way that gal moved.

Thank god for TV; it makes up for not being able to get out as much."

After he completed his apprenticeship and established himself at the *Times*, Lev married Sonja, they had a son, Michael, and a daughter, Raisa, and bought a one-family home, a first for his family. He had to moonlight to meet expenses—making jewellery and doing professional photography, mostly weddings and graduations. He often wondered "whether it was worth it for a lousy $1,200 a year" but sees now that being an entrepreneur forced him out of himself and let him meet artistic people. And he still enjoys the memory of "telling all those rich people where to stand. I'd seen what a good education could give you; rich people could afford to buy jewellery and have their photographs taken."

Sonja died when she and Lev were both very young. Lev didn't tell me how (he never liked to "dwell on the past," preferring to "stay in the present"), but it was a "watershed, it taught me to accept the impermanence of everything. Before, I was living like a grasshopper. Now I have two things I say about anything that happens: 'Will it change my way of life?' And 'This too shall pass.' With her death, something went out of me forever." Although he still had all his old friends, a piece of him "turned off, so that even now, after all these years," he has what he calls a bad character trait. He can have a very warm relationship with someone for years. But if he's "scolded, the only way I can explain it to you"—he snaps his fingers—"In my *mind*, I call it switching off. In a matter of minutes, I lose all feeling for them, just as if they've been dead for 20 years or never existed. It bothers me, not so much because I've lost something, but because I feel like a lousy bastard." By "scolded," he means that he doesn't like being told he isn't living up to someone else's expectations unless it's in a painting class, where he's there to learn, his work is respected, and there's no pressure to agree with the critique—where he can "take it or leave it, and no hard feelings."

Lev married a second time. He and Riva moved closer to family and friends—six couples met every week to play cards. When his father died, his mother, who lived a few blocks away, had time to see more of her grandchildren and shared with them her love of music and her stories of the old country and their hard early years in the United States. She nursed Riva during a long illness and helped Lev raise his children after Riva died. "I'd have been lost without her," he says.

His mother is dead now, Raisa died three years earlier of leukaemia, and Michael is in Alaska, "which is OK. He's an engineer up there and a good kid, but we have nothing much in common now except fishing. Those were my best times with him, but I can't fish anymore, now that my ticker is winding down." Old friends are dead or have moved away, except for one couple with fewer health problems than he has, "but they are so panicky, they might as well put on a wooden overcoat [coffin]. My painting gang is all out in Long Island, and I don't see them as often. So it goes."

A New Life

Just before Lev retired at 62, a friend suggested that he give up photography and jewellery making to paint. "She nagged me into to it, and it's the best thing that ever happened to me in my life, I took to it like a gull to the air. It opened up a whole new world for me." Some of the people he'd met in art class had painted on the island, and they persuaded him to drive them all up in his old jalopy—trading the ride for gas money. One week became two and now it's three—more would "break the bank." Every year he takes a class from one of the summer painters, and over the years he's painted on every trail, in every type of weather. Now, with his body "as crocked up as my old rust bucket," these same friends drive him and he pays for gas and buys lunch. "These are my best times now," Lev says. "I look forward to coming here the day after I leave."

His son paid for his three weeks on the island for several years, until, to his great surprise, Lev began to sell paintings. Most of the other artists have regular studio hours on specific days, but Lev never does—he doesn't want to be tied down to a schedule—no more unwanted responsibilities. His work hangs on the walls of his room and out on the porch, and when he's there he shows visitors around; when he's away, they can go in and look. There is never a missing canvas, and if someone walks off with one he'd "take it as a compliment, someone wanted a painting so much." Eventually word got around, and he was asked to exhibit at the Island Gallery. When I congratulate him, he shrugs self-deprecatingly, "Oh, well, maybe it's because people got tired of me not being there when they came."

Lev never dreamt that anyone would pay money for a painting, let alone one of his. So he gave them away until he realized that "painting was like carpentry, or any other work, and deserves to be paid for." Then he thought the people who bought his canvasses "must be crazy, or not know anything about art." He'd see the work of well-known artists from Boston, New York and Rockland in their island studios and feel like such an amateur that he "was ashamed to show his face behind an easel." Eventually he made enough sales to pay his own way and didn't have to "be dependent on his son's charity or anyone else's. So I could see it was going to be useful, and I kept on. But it's still strange for me to call myself a professional artist, and not just another Sunday painter."

Although the amount of money people pay for a painting still surprises him, Lev has discovered the "vanity" of the art market; the more he charges, the more people seem to want the painting—his range from $150 to $800. He also discovered some of the petty jealousies success can bring; one day he found that Sally, the manager of the hotel, had removed his roadside studio sign; her husband was a landscape painter. "I guess she thought I took away from her husband's sales," he says, "but we're completely different. Anyway, he thinks my stuff isn't any good, because it isn't 'true to nature.' And some people say I change my style too often. But I want to experiment with different styles, not get bogged down doing the same thing over and over, the way some artists do." He looks at me sideways, grinning when he sees that I agree, "I guess I'm still on the fringe."

Painting What He Feels

Lev says that the way he paints expresses his personality; the exuberance in the picture *is* him. "I know I'm like my painting—and it's like me." He will have a response to something he sees or about a remembered image—ocean, sea birds, fishermen, lovers—and then the work "comes right out of my gut. I squeeze my eyes shut and try to feel like a wave, or a lonely gull sitting by itself on a rock"; he points to a painting of a gull looking down at the waves washing over the rock it's sitting on. Then he gestures towards a nude on the other wall of his room: "With that one, I wanted to get the feeling of a heavy person feeling as light as a feather."

"She does look like that," I say; "she looks very pleased with herself, too. Now those two women in that painting over there, sitting in the sand dunes with their backs to each other, they look like they've had an argument."

"You got it. You've no idea how long it took me to get that tit just right!"

"You mean sort of—alert?"

"Yeah," he laughs. "Every breast I ever touched I remember as if it were yesterday. I know exactly what I want the painting to feel like, and I have no idea what it will look like when it's finished. I remember going out with a painter friend, and she painted all the details, the leaves on the trees, every blade of grass. I just sketched the essence, the feeling is the essence; I painted it years later. I could give you a story for every painting; each one comes about in a specific way."

Lev's paintings *are* very different from both the representational and abstract work on the island (or anywhere else, for that matter): bold shapes, vivid colours, and striking patterns that hang together so incredibly well that they have an immediate, and irresistible, sensual appeal.

I comment that he describes the way he paints in the same way that he's told me how he remembers events: once he has a key word, he sees the scene as if it's unrolling right before his eyes, and then he picks out the details he wants. In painting, his gut reaction to what he sees or remembers is like a key word: it summons and organizes what he expresses on a canvas. He replies that I may have a point, although he's never thought about it that way, because he doesn't think painting is really about memory. "I'm experiencing something. The technique is learning *how* to express the feelings."

He never forgets the feelings that drove the paintings. "Once I remember, once I have the incident, or see where something was, they all come back as if they just happened." But the idea that memory is more than an intellectual process, can live anywhere else but in his mind, still bothers Lev. One day we were having a conversation with Meyer and Miriam, long-time summer residents. Lev was stoutly maintaining that he made sketches from his imagination, "and that isn't memory." Meyer asks him how he does this.

"Well, I think about how a fisherman looks, how he feels when he is casting a line, and will experiment in the sketch until I get the line of the shape I am picturing."

"So you are *remembering* that, how he looked, how he felt?" Meyer asks.

"Yes, but it's not *just* memory. I remember how he looks, and I am feeling it when I am painting it."

"So, you put it together, some image you remember, and when you're remembering it, the feeling comes up, as if you were there." (Meyer was relentless when he wanted to track something down.)

"As if I were there *now*," Lev insists. "It's a two-way street. Whether I am remembering it, or when I am right there seeing it, it speaks to me in the same way: I feel it, and then I try to express it, to paint it."

"So, it's like you have a mind memory and a gut memory, they both bring out feelings that you paint," says Meyer, and Lev throws up his hands, saying he doesn't really care what anyone calls it, he'll keep on painting the essence, wherever it comes from.

I laugh whenever I come into my living room and see Lev's painting of the two women sitting on the beach, reliving his exuberance. The one of fishermen hauling nets into a boat, the sleeves of their oilskins covering their hands, hangs in my breakfast room. One day I'd asked him why he never painted hands, and he laughed, telling me that he can't make hands look the way he wants, so he finds a way to leave them out: ever the iconoclast. "Rocks I can paint, but not hands," he says, "because I can imagine how a rock feels, standing there alone, heavy, hardly able to move—although they do move, the geologists say, even breathe, and the waves change them, over a long time." With hands, it's a matter of a technique he's never mastered, because he's preoccupied with getting the line of the shoulder and of the arms straining as they pull in the weight of the nets.

"You can feel that straining?" I ask him.

"Oh, yes, I've done plenty of fishing; I know just how it feels in my arms and shoulders. You can't forget that kind of thing."

A Little Forgetting Beats the Alternative

Lev readily acknowledges that he forgets more than he used to. He knows that his medication affects his memory for details; the doctors warned him about the side effects—"a little forgetting is better than not being here." He's nonchalant about it, because he's never bothered to remember details that aren't useful anyway.

"It's like kids cleaning a blackboard: adults have erased the clutter so many times, things get forgotten. For an older person, there's a lot in the pot, and if you don't use something, you forget it—like now, I forget the conversion table for silver I knew when I was making jewellery. I don't care about that anymore."

Lev attributes other kinds of forgetting to sudden changes, or to habit, not to age. For example, he lives in a poor neighbourhood where there are a lot of break-ins, so he hides his valuables "in places that not normally, under no circumstances, would I put them, and then, by golly, I can't find them: that's not age." I tell him that I do the same thing. He looks satisfied—"and you're young"—and tells me about his lifelong bad habit of forgetting names and sometimes appointments if he doesn't write them down. It never used to bother him, but now it embarrasses him—such as when he forgot our appointment for lunch, "just as if it had never existed."

"Well, I came up and found you," I remind him.

"And we begged some lunch from Nancy [the cook at the hotel] and had a good time," he smiles, "just like we usually do. Anyway, I think there must have been a time when I talked myself into forgetting names, or I didn't really care, thought it wasn't important. Now it's a handicap, like a club foot, because people's names are important to them, and they get angry if you forget them. One time I solved the problem by making a big sign: HANDICAPPED PERSON WITH MEMORY FORGETS NAMES, and walked around with it on the road. Everyone laughed and forgave me. Someone took a picture."

"I could use a copy of that, hang it on the wall in my office!" I say.

"I don't know if I remember who took it," he laughs, "but if I do I'll send you one."

What troubles him more: deafness affects his ability to follow a discussion. "I don't think it's my mind, it's not being able to hear everything that is being said where the talk is rapid and several people are speaking at once. Phone conversations are worse: when you have a hearing aid, listening to people's voices is like mixing colours in a funnel, all the voices sound the same, which affects my memory, because there is no way to differentiate the voices and know who you're talking to."

As Meyer said, "senses are senses, they're all related." *Now that I wear a hearing aid, I understand: music has lost some of its character, and indistinctness over the phone affects my image of people, as well as what I hear them say.*

Swan Song

These kinds of forgetting were minor details for Lev compared to his heart condition and its increasing effects on his mobility, which he found suffocating. It depressed him so much that, although he has hated hospitals and doctors ever since his wife and daughter died, he finally agreed to a coronary bypass after a friend's had given him a new lease on life. Lev had high hopes, but the operation was only partially successful. He still has to take diuretics and other medications, still can't walk far, particularly in cold weather.

When we meet the next summer, we talk about his being "confined to barracks." However, never one to dwell on his feelings, he mentions some compensations, such as reading more selectively.

"The quality of the writing has to be faultless, otherwise I can't concentrate. I give the book about 50 pages, and if it doesn't pull me on, I go get another one."

"That seems like a fair enough test at anytime," I respond. "There are a lot of books to read."

"And there's no point in wasting time on ones that don't hold your attention," we chorus together.

Since the bypass, Lev can't paint as much so is surviving on his old age pension—poor once more, and more alone than he ever thought he could tolerate. He considers himself not old, but poor and disabled: when he starts to do something and can't continue because of heart pain, he becomes acutely aware of his "undependable body" and "fewer financial resources." He wonders constantly whether his life is worth living anymore—he accepts that his body is deteriorating and that he must "plod along with what remains," but there is the ever-present question of "to be or not to be?"

"It's a distraction. It's not the pain, and I am not afraid of death. When it's over, it's over, and I've come close enough to think of it as a relief. But in the back of my mind, I'm preoccupied with making a decision—it's like living with a voice in the next room asking whether I want to put up with the quality of life I have now. That voice is taking up so many grooves in my mind that there's no room, it's blocking out things, it affects my memory. But that's not the worst fear."

His worst fears, he reports, are intellectual decline and restrictions on his physical mobility. He knows that medication, not deafness, causes most of his cognitive problems; but it still worries him, because when he can't read with his old concentration, he finds it hard to keep from thinking that it's his "mind that's going downhill." The other fear is being unable to go out and meet people or go to the opera and ballet. He is "back in the cheap seats" and climbing stairs, which is becoming next to impossible. And he's desperate to be able to go out because he thinks he can never paint at home, alone. "Anyplace I can walk on the level, I walk. But if I can't get out and walk, if I can't move around, going to different places, because it requires physical exertion—for me that's a vital part of what I need. Absolutely vital. If I can't get out, I won't have the quality of life I want, and if I don't have the quality of life—that's it. I'm out of here."

Already experiencing the effects of early degenerative disc disease (*and even more sympathetic now in my own older age with damaged knees and creaky bones*), I ask him how he's managing. He tells me that his doctors say the only way to deal with not being able to get going in the morning is to wait. "They don't know why, but it takes a 'sort of awakening to get the juices flowing again.'" He finds that if he goes right out, he can't walk more than two blocks, but if he's active in the house for an hour or so, and then goes out, he has fewer problems. "So something has to start flowing again."

"It's not conserving energy, is it?" I ask.

"No, no," he says, "it's … it's like *letting* it come up, not forcing anything. It's like being groggy in the morning when you didn't have enough sleep, and taking longer to wake up. You can't push that, it just has to happen." But he still wonders about what he'll do when he hasn't enough energy to do what he wants. One time he was so depressed that he thought he "was coming to an end" and gave away all his possessions. But he missed music so much that he bought a Walkman and some tapes and found that the earphones compensated for his hearing loss just enough for him to be able to enjoy music again. Whenever there's an obstacle, Lev looks for ways around it, but the obstacles to finding people to paint with were becoming harder and harder to overcome.

I missed going to the island for a few years. Lev and I called each other and then wrote letters when his hearing made phone chats impossible. The summer he was 80, he couldn't manage the hill to the dining room without at least three nitroglycerines and a helping hand. His favourite waitress offered to take him meals when he couldn't make it until Sally objected that it took too much time. So he invited everyone to come and visit him; they brought food, and they picnicked together in the cottage living room, sometimes with a fire in the old grate.

Although he couldn't go out with them anymore, he took part in the painters critique at the end of the day and in a group show at the Island Gallery. That led to a one-man show at the art gallery in Rockland, and then the Island Gallery invited him to be one of its permanent artists, which made him "feel humble and grateful at the same time, but that's it for me on the island. This is my last summer. I feel as if the show at the Rockland is my swan song."

Sudden Renaissance

But Lev had a surprise coming. In his next letter: "I am amazed at how my painting is improving all the time. I've been functioning very poorly and have not been moving around so much, so have been doing more painting. All these years I've never been able to paint when I'm at home alone. My painter friends visit me, and we look at what I'm working on, but we can't paint together, there's not enough room to swing a cat. But being housebound and alone so much, my deterioration has had a beneficial effect by my starting to paint when at home! All there is left to do is paint.

"And surprisingly, as my body keeps falling apart and rotting, my painting is improving by leaps and more leaps— and it amazes me that while I can hardly work for more than 20 minutes without getting pooped, my painting is zooming, both design-wise and colour-wise, the feelings come pouring out. With every gain there's a loss and contrariwise. I haven't enough energy to carry a half a gallon of milk, but I can still push a brush around, and I'm able to achieve on canvas more than ever the concepts—scenes, people etc.—I have in my head.

"I blame it all on my four or five joke books. Every time I smell I'm going down I reach for a book and a few laughs puts me on the up elevator again. 'The surgeon general has determined that being alive makes one susceptible to many problems,' and I'm sure getting my share. Another show at the Rockland, and The Island Gallery wants more. Not sure if I can keep up, but I'll keep on doing it until the brush gets so heavy I can't push it anymore."

In his last letter to me, Lev said that it was becoming even harder to paint. "I don't have anything here I don't need, but I've warned my friends to go to my apartment as soon after I kick the bucket as they can, because the place will be stripped before you know it. I don't blame them, they're poor, and I won't be needing anything in my wooden overcoat. My friends have all my paintings except the one I'm working on now."

Lev died, brush in hand, of a massive coronary. Thirty artists hosted "A Tribute to Lev Bronsky" at the National Art League in New York. His paintings are big sellers on the island and in galleries on the east coast and in New York. But mine won't leave my walls.

Brush In Hand

The sea crashing against the old shipwreck
his "juice of life,"

a meal around the table his friends unspooling
the thread of an argument,

sunset livid on the rocks by the schoolhouse—
where evening dancers laugh,

in the thick of the day's critique with painters
hard at it by the light of a coal-oil lamp.

Alone and ill, brush in hand, canvases
fill with life until

his heart stills.

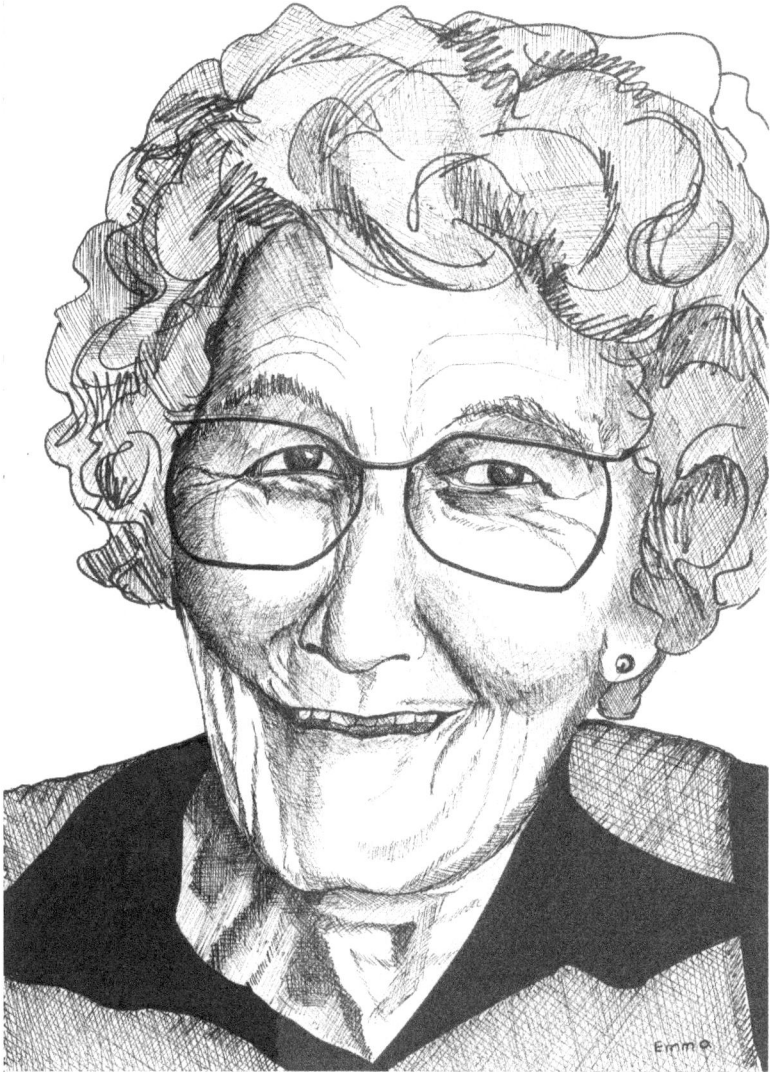

Coming Home: Emma's Story

"Dismiss the impossible, accept the inevitable and take on a new interest."

Life in Two Worlds

Fingers tap the sharp clop of horses' hooves as the carriage approaches, the sensuous silk of her father's hat brushes her knee as he doffs it: "Sit still, darling." Perching on his shoulder, she holds tight around his neck: "Sit still; you're going to see the Queen, the Queen of England." The old Queen's frail, black-gloved hand waves acknowledgment to the people cheering her Diamond Jubilee as Emma waves her own hand with a soft, faraway look, remembering waving at the Queen when she was two years old.

"And I did. I saw the Queen in her horse-drawn coach. I remember all the way back. An actress friend of mine said that if I can do that, I must have total recall." Emma continued:

> You see, everything has a sound,
> a picture: I can hear
> the clucking of my mother's chickens
> riding on the roof
> of the carriage on the way to
> our new home in Sheffield. It was
> the one possession she insisted
> on taking,
> And that parrot!
> We were visiting my uncle's house
> in Liverpool, the grandest house I'd
> ever seen. I came down early
> in the morning to look at the piano,
> the green silk behind the fretwork

of the music stand, and
silver candlesticks at either end.

Then a loud voice shrieked: "Damn you,
get out." Terrified I rushed out
right into my uncle's arms. "Don't be
frightened, darling," and he carried me over
to the long mahogany curtain rod to
look at the bird, but I reached out, and it bit me.

She showed me the scar on her thumb.

Sitting around the table for the last time before they left for Canada, her father fetched the Bible and, letting it fall open ("That was the custom at the time"), read the first verse on the page: "Be not afraid for I will be with you wheresoever thou goest."

"This was a prophetic verse for my family. We had years and years of poverty and hardship, and whenever my mother felt downhearted he would quote it: 'Don't worry, Mary, remember that verse.' And I always have: when I'd used up all my savings looking after my brother (there was no OHIP [Ontario Health Insurance Plan] then, you know), after my husband died intestate, I was almost 70 and only the house was mine, so I kept house for my nephew's family. When my grandnephew was in school, and they didn't need me anymore, I nursed, cleaned houses, and babysat. I gave music lessons until I was 80."

Music has been Emma's lifelong joy. A strong, vibrant thread running throughout her life, it provides meaning and continuity, context and connection, a loving memory web weaving together the cloth of past, present, and future. A springboard to a wide variety of personal and professional interests, it is also a link to family, friends, and community, a means to earn a living, and an enduring comfort and companion.

I was a year old when I heard
the negro minstrels at
the seaside and hummed all their songs;
my parents weren't musical,
but they decided I must be
and made music a part
of my education (at great
financial sacrifice). We two girls
were given the same
education as our brother,
which wasn't usual, you know.

I had music lessons at the
Conservatory from the time I
was 14. My teacher was a
woman of zeal who loved music,
children, and teaching and
encouraged me to take music seriously.

"Almost from the start," Emma recalls, "I made up my mind I would have music for a career and practised after school every day, tried my ACTM with musicians who later became well-known. They recommended me for a teaching position. I taught for 30 years at the Conservatory and met so many people who became good friends. Some of them are still alive, like me; they're not well off either, you can't be, without a pension, or considerable put by."

For Emma,

Music comes unbidden; I will wake
in the middle of the night with
the sound of a concerto or a fugue
playing. I listen, maybe sing
a little, and then go back to sleep.

There was music on board the ship
Lake Ontario *(a Cunarder,*

not like the poor Titanic*),*
mornings when we sipped consommé
and again at dinner. One day
I heard someone playing an accordion,
just like the minstrels,
and peered over the railing to see
people eating fish from a barrel
with their hands, and a little girl waved.

In the dining room, they ate
corn on the cob with their hands,
which upset my mother,
until she learned that it was
a custom of the country (like eating pears
without a knife and a plate).
We learned to like corn on the cob
very much—but I still like a plate
for a pear, if it's a good one.

The ten-day crossing was exceedingly happy for Emma. The family was all together, which wouldn't happen again for a long time, because her father's job involved a lot of travelling. She remembers her mother looking beautiful in grey broadcloth and her brother's pride in his first pair of long pants. They didn't often have new clothes.

Our first night in Canada turned out
to be very frightening.
A friendly professor on board ship
offered us lodgings with his widowed sister.
It was dark, I took my brother's hand
to go up the long, gloomy stairs and went to
sleep on a cot at the foot
of my parents' bed. In the middle
of the night, we started up to
the sound of a man's deep voice. Poor
woman, she read her late husband's speeches

at night, imitating his voice
for comfort.

The professor was apologetic
but we had to go somewhere else.
Since it was the clergy
you went to if you were in trouble,
we went
to the local Anglican minister,
who found a good place for us
with someone who needed the money
and was glad of the company.

Haliburton and Adventures

For almost 40 years Emma spent as much time as she could at her cottage in Haliburton. She and her father built it together—she learned to be a competent carpenter and electrician and could fix just about anything. I knew Emma when I was a young woman, and I have wonderful memories of Cranberry Lake: watching the lines in her face smooth out as the energy poured into old bones when we neared the lake (just as happens for me now, when I approach water), awestruck as she negotiated the road down to the shore over precipitous and slippery Precambrian shield. Emma's problems with her back and legs became so serious that she could no longer drive long distances. She taught me how to steer over and around those rocks, but it always seemed a perilous drive to me, sure that I'd drive straight into the water.

There are before-dinner drinks in front of the fire (just one—and a little dividend—so as not to stress her heart), short legs gratefully propped on a stool, iron-grey hair turning russet in the firelight, her round, plump face now dreamy and thoughtful, now animated, brown eyes alight, as she tells me stories of her life.

She loves visits with her friends from the music and art worlds who come bearing food, companionship, and "good talk." There are riotous conversations about the people and events of that world, such as the ones with Anna Russell, an opera singer and comedienne who is a deadly mimic and entertains us until the tears roll down our faces.

There comes a day when the rocky terrain is too much for Emma's unsteady legs. She would have liked her beloved cottage to stay in the family, but no one wants it, or can afford to buy it. (How I would have loved to, but, like her, I had no money to spare.) She tells me:

So I faced up to the fact that
I could no longer entertain
and decided that the best thing
to do was to wipe the slate clean,
sell it, and have enough money
to travel. Neighbours
had been waiting to add it to
their property. They invite me
to visit, but I won't go back,
no matter how much I miss it.

Instead I went to Monte Carlo,
"a sunny place for shady people,"
as Somerset Maugham said.

And I've been to places I'd always dreamt
of visiting and never thought to see.

Years ago I fell in love
with the poetry of Robert Service,
especially two verses about Alaska.
The image remained in my mind all of
my life, and I resolved: "Someday I'm
going to Alaska." Well, it had to be,
when I reached my ninetieth year
I thought,
"If I don't go now, I may never."

I sailed on the ship Rotterdam *(a Cunarder)* —
eight days of wilderness
and snow-capped mountains
and little ports where I met people
who came back, like Service did,
because they loved Alaska so much.

"Why do you suppose they loved Alaska so much?"

"Because they have no cares or worries; why would they, when there's nothing coming in from outside—it's like living on a ship. That was like living in a dream come true for me, the luxury of the liner ... my bed turned down every night and a Dutch chocolate wrapped in gold paper on the pillow ... and the magnificence of the scenery."

She described it all in lyrical, vivid detail: shapes, colours, sounds, textures, the population of towns, the height of mountains, the rate of glacial melt.

The glaciers were smaller than the ones
I saw crossing the ocean as a child,
when the Cunarder would anchor during
the night and move
not much faster than a man can walk.
It's a great privilege to live,
especially if you have your sight,
to be able to enjoy all the beauties of nature
and see, at 90,
the world as God must have made it.

When I ask her how she managed to get on and off the tender that took the passengers to ports on shore, she told me about Fred, who met her on the dock at the beginning of the voyage: "I had to put my age on a form, and they must have thought I would need special attention because I'm so old."

"Are you Mrs. P?" he said.

"I am."

"Good Lord, you're not 90! I've been told to look after you. This is going to be fun—and it's going to be easy."

They put us at Table 43
at the eight o'clock sitting.
When I told the others
how I came to be there, they
asked me to tell them the poems
of Robert Service.
Every night I recited one,
or a sonnet by Shakespeare, until
everybody got into it.

When we weren't on shore or taking part
in one of the shipboard
activities, we went fishing in
the ship's tender, and the chef cooked
our fish for lunch.

When Emma registered for a trip to the Caribbean, another place she'd always dreamt of seeing, "the first person I saw was Fred, who told me they'd called him when they saw my name, and he jumped at the chance. There I was, 91 years old, with a 70-year-old escort! We had fun. When I don't enjoy life, I don't want to live anymore."

Recipe for Success
Independence

As she tells me about Alaska, Emma recites the poems and sonnets she recited each evening at dinner. Occasionally she stops, calmly waiting for a word, or begins again, with no apologies, because she hasn't "done it properly ... I lose the rhythm. I remembered them better at dinner, but so much has happened since then to distract me. I had this crash, hurt my leg. I'm feeling quite ill. It's not age that affects my memory; it's the illness—it's distracting, it puts you off your beat. It's just that on some days you remember better than others. I think you do when you're 90."

Until lately she has just accepted that she doesn't remember names, never has, and never bothered to do anything about it. Now it embarrasses her, because, like Lev, she is more aware of how people like having their names remembered, and she is "now going out of her way to meet new people" [at 90, most of your friends and many relatives have died]. When a name gives her "temporary trouble," she will tell herself, "'It will come in a minute,' and it does."

"You seem to trust that it's there."

"That's right, I do. I have complete faith in my memory; when waiting a minute doesn't work, I leave it, wake up at three in the morning, and there it is! Like the writing on the wall. I have my ways, like a mental filing cabinet, of how people and places look, which registers in my mind the way patterns of sound do." (As they do for Meyer.)

Emma has passed her driver's test every year since she was 80, but she is making plans for when she can no longer drive (her car is her legs, as is mine). She needs a magnifying glass for the telephone book, and fatigue overtakes her "more quickly and more often than it used to, which is inevitable.

"But I don't worry, that would be useless. I rest every afternoon if I'm going out at night, groceries can be delivered for seniors, although I'll miss talking to people I meet—small towns are like that, you know. I've always said that the best way is to make a plan, and then forget about worrying, and I have designed a pattern for living for when I cannot drive. Like my 93-year-old friend who pays for help in the house when friends or relatives are too busy to come, and she buys concert and theatre tickets for herself and a friend who drives now that there's too much glare for her to drive at night. I have my cottage money, and so now I can do the same as she does and continue to stay happy and fulfilled."

"You plan ahead so you won't be taken by surprise," I say.

"No" (quietly), "changes won't come as a shock. And I can still go to England," which she still thinks of as her place of origin, her other home, and where she is passed around among the cousins' families (with whom she has corresponded all these years) like a treasured heirloom and where, while she is there, she runs the show. A somewhat frazzled cousin of 70 once told me, "Her vitality seems inexhaustible. She never shuffles along or is stooped, like so many very old people. Oh, she's a little stouter—and a little slower, but she carries herself just the way she always has. She plans each day to get the most of it and is quite testy with the Almighty when the weather is too hot for her body to do what the rest of her wants to do. But then she will always play the piano or settle down with a book."

"Independence of thought" is very important to Emma and encompasses both action and reflection—that is, doing what she wants to do and having "a good opinion" of herself, not "playing down my personality. I am not humble, but I'm grateful that things have turned out the way they have. It hasn't been easy. But then, women are better planners than men, and so they make better adjustments in their lives than men do.

"Most men are entirely absorbed in their jobs, few love the work they do; they work for the cheque to support the family, and their interest in life ceases beyond that point. When they retire, they are lost in dark days of pessimism. A woman is more selfish, she has a self-importance that doesn't belong to men. She thinks of herself as an important member of society.

"I've been to those groups where women sit around in a circle trying to convince themselves they're important. I have to hold my breath so I won't giggle. You don't need to be convinced of that, you know it, if you had any sense you'd know you're important."

"Why do you know you're important and these women do not?"

"Because I'm a child of God, and so are you, and so is everyone who is born."

"Paul says we are born in sin," I tease.

"Nothing of the kind," Emma retorts tartly. "I don't believe in the Immaculate Conception or that Christ was anything else than a person. But somebody created the universe—I call it God—so that everything keeps in its course, in the right place. You cannot put a hand on anything that God has not made. Do you know anything that has made itself?

"God is everything you feel inside; you can no more escape from God than you can escape from yourself. People wouldn't have to have these cults to feel their importance if they only realized why they were here. That's all that's needed. To me it's a plain and simple fact. Atheism is bad for your self-esteem."

I remember when I was ten years old,
walking out on the prairie from
the back door of the house—
and those days it was alone—nothing
between you and the horizon, wild crocuses
growing around the springtime puddles.
It came to me suddenly
what a wonderful thing God did
when he made the world. What a wonderful
thing He did when He made me. That I wasn't alone
and that I am a child of God. Everyone is.

"Christ must have been rugged to endure what he did. It was the Italian artists who made him soft and delicate—a terrible thing done to his name. His philosophy would have saved the world. It still could. It was Paul (I'm not very fond of Paul, I can tell you), a woman hater, who brought politics and power into it so that Christianity deteriorated to the point of the Inquisition."

Unhappy memories are as vivid to Emma as happy ones. In fact, according to her, the habit of "deliberately forgetting unpleasantness is the beginning of a bad memory." She doesn't forget them but doesn't "dwell on them," rarely talking in any detail about the hardships in her life, even to people she knows well. As she says (and as I've learned over the years), "No one wants to hear about your troubles; they just want to hear what's interesting to them." She has never discussed how she felt about having her nephew subsidize her or about his family, who had a place on a lake near hers, not helping her to keep the cottage. But I did know of their every exploit and triumph. They were her only family in Canada.

Like Rebecca, as she becomes older she "switches off violence" and makes a point of remembering only good, because, she says, the evil in the world is only a minority. "The great number of people the world over, what I call humanity, is concerned with marrying, family, keeping a roof over their heads, and having enough food. Those who are weak enough to indulge in crime I am not interested in. I don't want to know them. Just think of the thousands of volunteers who help people, including me."

Total Recall

"Oh, I can remember anything I want to anytime, it's a special gift, and I've treasured it all my life. Everything that happens to you is in your subconscious, which we all have, only it can lie dormant when no demands are made upon it. Only people with total recall have the ability to bring it to the surface verbally. People who say they have a bad memory just talk themselves into it. They make no demands on their mind."

When she wants to remember something, she will think back to where she heard it the first time, what the person looked like, the surroundings. She "has a gift for remembering every detail of a person's home. I could make you a list of pictures, furniture, ornaments. I don't try to do that, it just registers in my mind."

"So you have a good visual and auditory memory?"

"Yes, very. Sounds … music … are a pleasure for me … I suppose it's love, a form of love which has me remembering."

For Emma, the whole purpose of life is to keep mentally alert, and the only way she knows to do that is to have a vital interest. She never has to "improve" her memory because she always has "a little more than I can do."But I'm kind to my mind. If something is too worrying, I put it aside and come back to it. As you get old, your energy declines, that's inevitable, so I don't fritter it away but use it only to a comfortable point. But lazy minds, that's appalling! I have young neighbours who sleep till noon on weekends. They miss so much, they never see the trees and birds in the light of early morning.

"Maybe they had lazy parents. Energy is something that's inherited, a constitutional vitality. My parents were very energetic and worked hard. They took long walks even when they were old. Now I can't do that, I have bad legs (all that standing when I was too old for it), but I always have something to do."

Like all the elders I talked to, Emma knows that you live more intensely as you get older. And like Meyer she is adamant that there are two ways of looking at this: "there's loss—the older you get, the more loss there is: friends, family, job, the places you can visit, what your body can do. But then there's experience; the old have an advantage over the young: every year you live you gather experience, and so your interests expand, because when you can't do what you're used to, you do something you can and might never have thought of. It's important to make up your mind at an early age to fill your life with things you can do, not with what you can't do. I'm working on my autobiography, and I can travel, now that I've sold the cottage."

Engaging with the Community

Emma volunteers in many different sectors. She founded the first seniors' residence in the town she lived in that provides continuous care, from townhouse, through assisted-living apartment, to full end-of-life nursing care. She writes a seniors' column for the local newsletter, sits on numerous social service and arts boards, is active in garden clubs and local animal rights groups—to name a few. One night over dinner I mentioned that I'd heard that the new auditorium at the residence was to be named for her. She would never have told me herself—that would have been boastful—but was pleased when I asked if there would be a dedication ceremony. She thought there'd be "some kind of party" and would let me know. She did, it was a very good party indeed, and it was heart-warming to see so many friends and appreciative, knowledgeable well-wishers surrounding her. A year later she received the Order of Canada for her service to the community.

When she reached 90 (which she had never expected to do, because her parents had died much younger), Emma said that she could think of herself as an old woman of many years of experience, which gave her a "certain authority" on quite a few subjects. In her opinion, the causes of a poor memory are indifference, fear, loneliness, and boredom, which must all be "deliberately avoided all of one's life because they have a debilitating effect on the mind." Everything that happens to you must be deliberate, because indifference is a "dangerous habit."

She talks about indifferent parents whose children become delinquent because they have not been brought up with "loving rules." And indifferent children who put their parents in an old age home "forget about them and condemn them to loneliness because they are afraid of the old, afraid to see what they will become, afraid of death … which is inevitable, so there's no point in being afraid."

Emma believes that tomorrow's elderly women, who will have had the education to find good jobs (as she did, but that was unusual then), will have interests to sustain them. But of her generation, most have been housewives; when their children leave home, "unless they have been readers of books," they are lost, and, like the forgotten old, are lonely and bored. Since people with no interests need others to stimulate them, these women, if they are smart, will take up community work, using their homemaking and child-rearing skills to serve someone else. "It's the only way I know to continue for anyone left alone, to become happy and feel that their life is fulfilled."

Times are not easy, and she knows she has to "continue to make adjustments." However, aches and pains, disability of legs and heart pale in comparison to her increasing deafness— "the greatest tragedy that has ever befallen me." She doesn't think deafness has anything to do with aging because "young people are deaf too," and she develops strategies to stay active in the community. She talks face to face with people and meets with smaller groups. Board meetings are fine—only one person talks at a time, and she always gets the minutes afterwards. I ask her if deafness has affected her memory, and she doesn't think so. "If anything, it sharpens your memory, you have a better grasp of the meeting after reading the minutes, because it's shortened down ... I study them thoroughly." She doesn't worry about having a rest during coffee break—"there's too much noise to hear anything anyway, and besides, people think I'm wonderful to still be able to make a contribution and don't think anything of it."

Sage Counsel

Emma was the first older person with whom I'd discussed memory and aging in any depth, and I was looking for her insight into how to coax people who didn't know me as well as she did to open up about themselves. Her memories seemed to come effortlessly, perhaps because we were at ease with each other. "What about people who may be feeling apprehensive?" I ask.

> *Ah well, these are the lost and lonely ones —*
> *their friends gone, their families indifferent,*
> *their interests few. They are left with nothing*
> *to do, and their vitality and memory ebb away.*
> *But those memories are never really forgotten,*

just unused, and will come back with careful
nurturing.

As she describes how to do this, her body quietens; face intent, brown eyes with an opaque, gazing-inward look to them:

All you have to do is say: "Where did you go to
school?"
and something works in the mind, takes them
back to the schoolhouse; there's hardly anyone of
any age who can't remember where they started school.
And then you say: "What was your teacher like,
was she nice, or not?" That leads from one thing
to another, and gradually you're getting them a little
older, a little older, until you say: "Now then, when
you left public school, what did you do?"
"Oh, well, there were chores on the farm, my father
was a farmer." "Is that so, did you have cows or what?"

You get all that out of them, and that takes quite
a while at first. And then you're off!
You can't ask them directly about memory.
It must be done in a much more subtle way,
as I've just described. Then you see
how their memories work, see at what point
they begin to forget, and then,
when you get home, you can draw your own
conclusions. And write an article on it, if you want to.

How Long to Live?

Several years later, at 95, Emma reports that her body, plagued for years with back, leg, and heart problems, seems to have suddenly fallen apart. She can no longer "manage" the meetings that "sharpened" her memory and is becoming increasingly dependent on home-care workers—"nice women, doing a hard job [she knows, she used to do it], but there's a different one almost every time, and so you can't discover what you might have in common."

She can no longer compensate for her deafness; it's much harder to summon the energy to go out to meet and talk with small groups or take part in board meetings. There are fewer friends who can visit and none who can drive to concerts, and—"the last straw"—her sight is beginning to fail: "I can't hear a word in church. The new prayer book is ugly, I can't follow it—I can't read the fine print, so I have no means of learning it and remembering it. So I've stopped going to church, and I won't be visited. That's not what I need. I'm not an invalid. I want to be able to take part, and there's no longer any way to do so."

I had an image of Emma sitting alone at a family party, that inward expression on her face, and my going over to talk to her and finding that she ignores the conversations she can't hear and "thinks of something else" until someone arrives.

Remembering that she'd said, "it's the clergy you go to when you're in trouble," I ask her if she'd talked with her clergyman about having big-print prayer books and hearing aids in the front pews, and she replies, "Well, I don't think that will do any good."

I was feeling badly for her, and sad. Over the years she had memorized the church service, which she loved for its familiarity, its language, its music, and the many associations she had made. Without asking her permission, I called on her minister, who listened and then said that he had "no idea of the extent of her difficulties" and would do what he could. "It's a matter of money, and there are so few people who need ..." he trailed off, not looking at me. I was glad I hadn't told her I'd called; she was quite right that asking wouldn't do any good. No wonder she was angry. I was angry for her, and suddenly feeling my own aging and what that will mean as she tells me:

> *I can't play the piano, but*
> *I can still listen to music. I won't*

hear all of it, but I will hear it in my mind.
I don't read much anymore,
but I can still recite poetry (mostly to
myself; there aren't too many
who have been brought up to enjoy it).
I can still envision all that I saw
in my travels and enjoy nature. When
I can't get out, I watch the birds at the feeder.

Emma was not to die in her house. When she was 97, the family and the home-care workers decided that her "disability was too great" and moved her (*she* didn't move) to the seniors' residence she had helped build, whose auditorium was named after her, but where she had thought she "would never live."

While she was still fighting the decision, I asked her if she had thought of selling an option to purchase on the house so that she could afford the additional help she needed to be able to stay there.

"There's no one to arrange it."

"Your lawyer?" (I'm struggling, too).

"No, there's not enough help. The family is very busy, and my younger friends are in their late 80s or 90s now and in the same boat. It's hard for people to keep me in their minds."

What she doesn't say, because she never allows herself "to dwell on unpleasantness" (or to acknowledge the "downside" of her feistiness), is what I discover on making inquiries. She has become angry, querulous, and demanding, the available help don't stay long and fewer people want to come. The kind of anger some old people have that often attracts attention—even negative attention is better than none[1]—works "only to a certain point," as Emma herself might

---

[1] Dr. Barbara Myerhoff, *Number Our Days* (NY: Touchstone Press, 1980). Based on her anthropological research: a portrait of a community of eastern European Jews in Venice, California—disadvantaged but resilient people sustaining their cultural heritage in poverty and loneliness in the modern United States.

have said. After that, "you are beyond the pale, and they get rid of you," as Russell does say.

The Voice of Aging

One of Emma's life sayings that I and my family remind each other of when life gets chaotic and confusing is "Plan ahead—then change won't come as a surprise." She met adversity by continually reframing what well-being meant for her, what was worthwhile, enjoyable, workable, meaningful—and memorable—to make the "best life possible under the circumstance." Did she ever think she would live so long that her plans would be ignored or unworkable, and her memories unknown?

Although the Order of Canada hangs framed on the wall with her family pictures, the community she served for so many years has grown old too, and there is almost no one left who has known that "wonderful, feisty old woman." Fewer still who have read her column "Voice of Aging" in the community newspaper with the header: "Dismiss the impossible, submit to the inevitable and take on a new interest."

Her angry rebellion against the extent of the impossible and inevitable is not seen as "feisty"; it "turns people off"—as she had foreseen about others. Caregivers have no fond memories of what she has meant to them to temper their impatience. There is no one left who is interested in her story, or who wants to listen—except her relatives. They have heard it time and again and know what is between the lines as she "deliberately selects from the past, and from the now," the memories she wants (can bear/bare) to remember, the memories she needs to talk about to maintain her well-being.

And so Emma lets go of expecting herself to be active and useful, the ways her society —and she—define "aging well," and turns inward to the sights and sounds that still give her pleasure. On my last visit she doesn't hear me at first when I knock on the door of her room. She is looking out the window at birds darting back and forth at the feeder, Chopin's

Ballade # 4 fills the room. Perhaps, as she did long ago at that family dinner, she is "thinking of something else until someone comes." Perhaps the sounds of nature and music are enough, "forms of love which have [her] remembering."

Coming Home

I did anything to support myself
and keep my house. I will die here.
I fell in love with it before I saw it
when I read about it. Warren and I
bought it, we married in our forties,
I was too old to have children, and he
had grown sons.

We raised cocker spaniels here
and kept Mallard ducks on the pond.
Plenty of fresh eggs. I had a place to teach
piano when I retired.

It's the only house I've ever
owned. I love my own bed and the
routine of the day, to set my place
in front of the window
so I can watch the birds and the
passing seasons. I never
thought to sell it when I needed
money.
Where would I come back to?

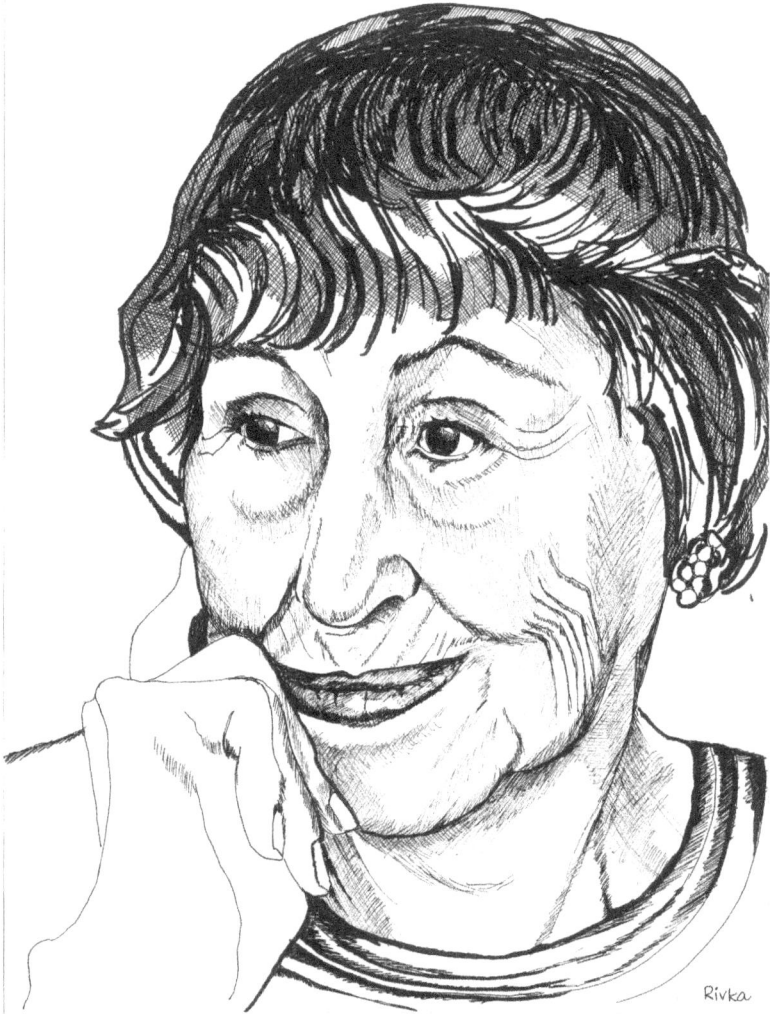

Rivka

The Heart of the Matter: Rivka's Story

"I feel myself so differently. I am better now. It's never too late."

I see her in a corner of the lounge at the Jewish seniors' centre in North Toronto: short, plump, grey-haired, sitting bolt-upright, hands folded on her lap, her face strained. She'd been in one of the workshops on memory strategies I'd given there and seemed pleased when I'd asked if we could talk later about her experiences. But when I phoned to arrange a time and a place, she hedged, and then was adamant that she didn't "want to talk about anything personal." Looking at her now, her tight smile as she sees me, I guess that my persistence is probably the only reason we are here.

During the memory workshop, the class had discussed lists of "What people tend to remember and forget" and Rivka relaxes a little when I ask her if she makes lists when she shops. She replies that now that she's retired and has more free time she doesn't have to. If she forgets a purchase one day, she can always buy it the next day and finds an alternative in the meantime.

"Does it concern you, when you have to do that?"

"Not really, it's just that I have a sister, we share an apartment, and I like to serve her needs, her preferences. That's why I have things on hand, and of course as you're entering the store you can look up at the signs and that reminds you."

"That's true, I do it myself all the time. Do you ever think much about memory?"

"No, I don't worry about it at all. My sister, though, she was an executive secretary and had to be right up to the mark. If she can't remember a word, it bothers her no end. I say, 'Look, no one is perfect, you don't have to remember everything right now, you're not working. If you forget it, it will come back to you later.'"

Bouncing Back

Rivka married when she was very young, "to have some sort of life." I don't ask so early in our conversation what she means, and she volunteers that her marriage had been "very good," but her husband died after 10 years, leaving her with a four-year-old daughter.

"I raised her myself, she's 39 now."

"With grandchildren?"

"No, I'm a mother-in-law, but not a grandmother. I love children. I miss being a grandmother. I don't envy people for the material things they have, I like more family things. However, maybe it's meant to be that way."

"Maybe it is."

As she veers away from missing grandchildren, I don't mention mine, who are such a joy, and ask where she worked when she was widowed.

"In a dress shop selling and helping with the buying. I detested it. It wasn't my cup of tea, I wasn't trained. I didn't have the necessary skills, and when my husband passed away, I had to take the lowest-paid, lowest kind of job. It was rough. That's why I'm on two high blood pressure pills a day. I try not to think about it; I'm glad it's behind me."

I see that we won't be talking about that for now—and ask if she enjoys retirement. She loves her leisure, she replies, but has to keep busy. When she was working, she hadn't time to do anything else except her job, housework, and caring for her daughter—"two jobs every day all day." When she first went to the seniors' centre, her "nerves were shot," and she knew she must work with her hands. She started with tiles and then went on to other arts and crafts—knitting, painting, clay. Now she enjoys the lectures more.

"You find you want more intellectual stimulation?"

"Oh yes, absolutely. Absolutely. Mind-expanding."

"Sounds like you needed some time—use your hands and just relax."

"That's right, that's right."

"Now you're kind of rested up from all that and feeling …"

Rivka hurried to say how much she likes the theatre: "We were laughing the other day, we had a gentleman here, Jewish, and he thought it was terrible we didn't get involved with Jewish theatre, as they call it. 'Well, you know,' I says to the others, 'one thing I could thank my mother for when we were children, she literally used to drag us off every Friday night—that was how I acquired a taste for plays—to the St. Lawrence Centre, or the Leah Posluns Theatre, and of course we had the opera tickets.'"

"Do you find you mostly remember the plays you've seen?"

"Ah, I don't always recall it all. It would have to be something that has meaning. Like I can never forget the movie *The Elephant Man*. I like anything to do with society, the treatment of people, and that has stood out in my mind so vividly."

I asked what operas appealed to her, and she said ones where the plot and voices are good, like *La Traviata* and *La Bohème*. She remembers some of the melodic arias and enjoys Luciano Pavarotti.

Of a movie about Mozart (*Amadeus*), she says she can't stand the way he was taken advantage of. "When there are people that are using other people, I just want to turn it off. Isn't that awful?"

"I don't think that's awful at all. Isn't that called a social conscience?"

"Possibly … but I just walk away from it … Maybe I don't do enough volunteer work, as much as I used to, now that I have more time to myself … I don't know why I don't."

I am treading carefully and don't follow up the link between social conscience and volunteering but take another path and ask her if it's because she wants to pursue her own interests. She agrees and tells me that she is still active at the centre and coordinates the Lifelong Learning program, where she introduces the speakers. Although she is thinking of taking a course on Speaking Confidently, she is already writing her own speeches and memorizes them until she knows them perfectly.

"And then, when I get to deliver it I'm afraid I'll get a block."

"You're afraid you'll forget it?"

"Yes. And I got my notes in front of me, and I think that reading from notes can be very boring to the audience. I try to look up; you must look up at your audience."

She has a pattern for her speeches and fills in the content appropriate to the speaker and the topic. Giving me an example, she forgets the speaker's name, looks upset and says in an exasperated voice, "So there, that's it you see. I'm still getting that block I've had all my life, even as a child at school we would have debates or discussions. I had it then."

"Possibly anxiety about …?"

"That's possible. I'm not seeing any senility up there, no way."

"I'm not either, not at all. It's that …"

"I want to do it right."

"And if you have been having this ever since you were a child …"

"Well, we were brought up in a very strict home."

"Were you?" *Cautiously, Ann.*

"Oh, yes. Yes, very. Not enough from the father, not enough encouragement. If you got a report, if your report was good—it could be 85 or 90—if there was a possibility of 100—not good enough. If you could cope with it, it was easy. Like my sister in between, she had a tougher skin and could handle it better. Now, I don't believe in false praising, but it has to be constructive. For me, it's not easy. Children will accept criticism sometimes from out of the home. At home, it has to be more praise. I don't know if I'm right or wrong about that."

"It certainly sounds like those were very high expectations."

"Maybe that's why I still want this perfection."

Too early to delve into the why, to risk crossing the line. At the beginning, we hadn't talked about what she meant by personal. Now I see a difference emerging between personal and private, but, since I'm not sure if it is she or I making the distinction, I continue, "And it makes you nervous that it's not going to be perfect."

"Right."

"You sometimes rehearse your speech before you give it?"

"I don't rehearse it, I memorize it. I can even say it right now, word for word. I have a first line—the first line is always the same." She recites a few lines, sits back, and smiles. "And it goes from there, depending on the topic of the day."

"Sounds good to me."

"That's the way I have to do it."

She changes the topic firmly, but not quite so abruptly, and I feel free to continue in the same vein, "Whatever works, eh? Do you ever have speakers about music, the opera? Sometimes the COC [Canadian Opera Company] gives lectures before the opera."

She goes for the music, can even sing along. With a chuckle, she tells me that once a woman near her was humming along, and people didn't like it. "Someone gave a loud 'Shush'—a lot louder than her humming—and she looked embarrassed. She hadn't realized anyone could hear her, she was enjoying herself so much. I sympathized ... You can do things without ... Anyway, that's OK."

She is steering us away again. I think I'm getting the hang of this.

"You remember the melody then. How do you do that? One musician I talked to said he remembered the personality of sounds, another, who is also a painter, said sounds have colour."

"Oh, yes—well, you hear them over and over. Just through memory, I guess."

"If you were to close your eyes and think back and say that you wanted to remember the aria from the first act of *La Bohème,* would you hear the sound, or visualize it, or ..."

"Well, it's not my favourite opera."

"OK, what's your favourite opera?"

"*Traviata* … or *Rigoletto* …" She sings a few bars of *Rigoletto*. "The others, they don't come out spontaneously, but the minute I hear them I try to associate, like you know, we have a little contest, my sister and I, to see which one we can remember."

"You remembered that one right away."

"Mmm. Spontaneously. Was I humming that before? I can't remember now." She sings a few bars of *La Bohème*.

"It may not be your favourite, but just now *La Bohème* came to you …?"

"Gives me goose bumps. It touches me."

"What happens? Are you feeling the sounds, and then …?"

"Feelings sounds, I don't quite follow that."

I ask her to try an experiment, to close her eyes and, as a piece of music comes to her, to observe what's happening. She sits with eyes closed for a minute, a little smile playing around the corners of her mouth, and then says, "Just by thinking."

"Just by thinking. And do you see anything, or is it a feeling kind of thinking?"

"More of a feeling."

It's not time yet to go into the feelings themselves but I say that it seems as if her feelings and memories are singing in her. When she first talked about writing a speech, she used the word "draw" and she's told me that she enjoys working with her hands. Now she is remembering music when it touches her, when she feels something.

Remembering Physically

"Sounds as if you're a kinaesthetic learner," I say to her. "One of the ways you learn is through your body, as well as your mind."

"Well, yes, I suppose I ... Well, hmm. Well, I don't know ... I'll have to think about that ..." She picks up the link to the aesthetic in kinaesthetic and says that she appreciates art and that in her spare time, when she first retired, she used to draw. But she thinks that a "real artist" has a more vivid imagination.

I follow her lead and approach remembering physically in another way and mention Alice describing to me how, in her early years as an artist, she had looked at a scene and remembered it through the rules she learned in art school— about form and motif and so forth. Over the years she's learned that she has to move away from rules to develop her own style.

Rivka looks down at her hands, "That's all right," she says.

I am pushing here. I have finally recognized that Rivka changes the subject when we move from the "what" of aging or memory—her practical strategies—towards the "how" in her body and emotions, and the "why" in her past.

She is thoughtful for a while and then tells me about a teacher in school who "favoured good drawers." So she learned to do it the way the teacher taught, recalled drawing imaginary lines that would meet at one point as a telephone pole, recollected drawing leaves. When she started art classes at the seniors' centre, she remembered those leaves and drew all the little lines and curves, differently for the elm and for the ash. She could recall the names of the species.

"And you'd remember ..."

"I'd remember, yes, and even now, I look for it—I look for nature. I love walking and the fresh air, I really do. Take that away from me, and I'm gone. This morning, I walked—I go for a walk every day, which I never used to be able to do—I call them my therapy sessions. I must get out in the morning and look around and have some time for myself."

She feels that when you are living with someone you must be away from each other sometimes. Then, when you return with renewed interest, you have something to talk about.

She doesn't have a TV and prefers radio. I said that I did too and observe that now she has time just to enjoy herself and the leisure to think about things.

"Well, that's it," she replies. "I was reading, but now I've gone back to newspapers again for some reason, you know you sort of go on and off things, don't you?" *Her first question to me.*

"Yes, you do. Do you remember the plots, the author's names? I have a hard time remembering names and titles."

"Pretty well. I'm interested in politics. I want to see what's going on in the world, current events, that sort of thing. I don't agree with what's going on in the world."

"International news?"

"Absolutely."

"What is socially meaningful, not the gossip columns or …"

"No, no. Sometimes the sports page (I watch hockey), not the obituary columns—some people do read those, you know," smiling at me for the first time.

"I know, I have a friend who says she reads them every morning to see whether or not she's in them." We are laughing together now.

"But I get browned off with the hockey because they start fighting with each other, and I can't stand that. I guess I'm a weakling or something, but, you see, it stays with me pretty well … always … It stays with me. But you can't help your feelings, and that's that."

We are getting pretty close to the personal, and she shuts off. But this time I don't have to fish around because she continues, "I find my powers of concentration have increased considerably since I've been taking the lectures."

Although the sudden change in topic throws me a little, "Has it?"

"Oh, definitely, definitely!"

She sounds very hearty—maybe a narrow escape? Or possibly she senses my temporary confusion. "Do you take notes during the lecture?"

"No, no, I don't, I listen."

"That's how you remember?"

"It depends on the lecture, what they have to say. If you've had a more extensive schooling, it's possible you would comprehend a little more. Like we have two lecturers coming here at the same time. One of the lecturers, we find we relate to her better—although she's a little bit of a hustler. The other, he sort of uses a little bit of jargon. I mean words that are only oriented to his profession and not what I call good English."

"Well, if you don't understand it, then I think you could call it jargon."

"Oh, I wouldn't say he doesn't know his subject, I give him credit for that, it's just that he thinks he's with his students."

This was the second non sequitur, and I was wondering if she had a slight hearing problem, so I continue about jargon and comment that it's so easy to slip into jargon and that my kids keep me on my toes: "Mum, you're using those words again," they say; "would you just say it in plain English?"

"Well, now, I did that once. I can't remember what lecture it was, it was a science lecture at a literary lunch, and I could see everybody had a blank face when we had a question-and-answer period. So I got up and said: 'Including myself, you'll have to go into more detail and more explanation, because we don't know what it's all about.' And she did. I wasn't enjoying her at all until she explained it in more detail."

"How did you feel—about getting up and … That took some chutzpah!"

"Oh, I felt fine—after I'd done it!—just fine. But, you know, we all have a feeling we don't want to show our ignorance and all that. It's like disagreeing with the doctor. I had to do that this winter, and I felt terrible. Doctors are right up there, you know."

"An authority—and we were brought up not to disagree with someone who's an authority—even when we don't understand!" I comment with some feeling.

"I guess we are. Pretty silly, when you come to think about it."

"Well, it's certainly … Where do you suppose that comes from?"

"Oh, I don't know, it's not really important now anyway."

Something that might bring up the past—but this time I acknowledge her reluctance and say that I think it *is* important *not* to think you're silly when you have feelings about what is important to you, and then invite her to go back to how she remembers. She says that if something has meaning for her, she'll concentrate, and then it will "get stored away … if it isn't important enough to stay in my mind, then it's not important." (Just as Callum said, "A moment's full attention is all that is needed.")

"How do you store it away? Some people repeat it, some people …"

"With my eyes and my head. My eyes store a lot." I love her practicality and asked her to explain.

"I'm looking at the lecturer, almost he is talking with his eyes to me."

"Un-huh, and then …"

"With my head—the information goes up there. That's where the brain is supposed to be," she says tartly. (*Oh good! Other than a few smiles, this is the first time she has shown her feelings.*)

"Right! You're not aware of any sort of repeating in your mind or …?"

"If it's a topic that I don't like, on TV or elsewhere, if there's cruelty in it or meanness, I feel it here," touching her stomach.

"You've said that then sometimes you'll block it out."

"No, I'll walk away from it."

"And if it's something that you like …?"

"I'm exhilarated."

"And where …?"

"All over. All over." *She sounds a little impatient now, as if I'm too slow in getting it.* "It's just like seeing the opera *Madame*

Butterfly. I've watched many, many productions, but about a year ago, at the O'Keefe [now Sony], it was the most beautiful production I've ever seen, especially the scene when the sun was setting and Cio-Cio San was waiting for Pinkerton. As she talks, she touches her heart: "Oh, the feeling, right here. How she watched and watched, and the sun was setting. And he didn't come ... That was ... I feel it now, just thinking about it. No part of me can forget it."

Body, Feelings, and Memory

I'm exhilarated. Rivka has been so leery about the personal/private, and here she mentions body, feelings, and memory in the same sentence. Not wanting to push I ask her if it has a social meaning for her as well.

"Oh, yes, when I associate it with a reason why. It's in my own background."

And glad I didn't push it. "The economic situation was very bad when we were children, problems of unemployment, strikes in Winnipeg—if you can remember."

"You lived in Winnipeg during the Depression? We were in North Bay, at the end of the railway line ... men coming back because they hadn't found jobs ... We didn't have much either, but my father was working, and my mother always had soup."

"Oh, yeah, so you know about that. So it may have something to do with it, or whether it just seems that you inherit it somehow. If you get that feeling—I hate to see anybody put down, like with Mozart. I just could not stand it. Couldn't stand what they were doing. Of course, it was partly his fault too, he was cavorting around, but it was sad ... horrible. I think maybe it's my background that may have indications for my feelings about these social situations."

"The kinds of things you grew up with as a child ... and then as a widow, bringing up a child on your own as a single parent."

"Exactly ... and not liking the type of work you are doing."

"Wishing you could find something else and regretting you didn't have other skills."

"That's right." Her sisters became confident secretaries, but, when she went to high school, an experimental curriculum was introduced. The students studied a wide range of 10—15 subjects, but they didn't focus on one subject long enough "so you knew what direction to go." She was supposed to be in the academic stream but it "wasn't enough. No, no, not enough, and not enough at home either, but that's all over and done with."

"And you're thankful for that."

"I am. Oh, I am!"

As I become more aware of when and how she changes the subject, I can go along with it more easily and this time turn back to daily living.

"We've talked about remembering what you're shopping for. Now …"

"Well, as long as I can get up and go and do my own shopping, I'm going to rely on my memory as much as possible."

"So you're saying as long as you can use your memory, as long as you're active …"

"Absolutely, absolutely. And when I'm reading actively, if I don't comprehend immediately, I'll reread until I get to the point of understanding."

"In a sense, that's a kind of practice, isn't it?"

She'll find what's "good for her"—that is, what suits her needs. For instance, when she first started visiting the seniors' centre, the staff asked her to take attendance at the lectures. She was going through a long list of names every week and got to know everyone's first names, and sometimes even their last names as well. After a while, she felt pretty good about herself.

"I guess it *is* all practice if you want to do something about it; if you're flexible about it, and say it doesn't matter when some people rush in and don't give you time. So now, I don't get irritated, the way I did in the dress shop, and rather than call them back, I just let it go."

"You have the intention, now you make it a point to remember."

"Absolutely, absolutely. And then I would encounter these people, and I would be able to say: 'Hello, how are you?' and use their first names. And I've gotten to like people a little better than I used to because ... oh well ..." *Her voice trails away,*

"Better than the people in the dress shop," I say gently.

"Yes!" she blurts out. "Do you know, I used to have to listen to all their stories about their illnesses, and, you know, when I first started here at the centre, if anyone came over to me and started talking about their sickness, I'd run away. I couldn't stand it. I had it close to 20 years in that shop—starting right after my husband died. And that's a lot. Then I attended a workshop here and learned a strategy. One of the ladies said: 'Well, I listen to my friends when they talk about it, whatever bothers them, but if some have a habit of going over and over it, that's it for me. I'll be sympathetic, I'll help them when I can, but I won't talk about it constantly. Forget about it for a while.' Now that *I* do that, I have a better rapport with people."

"Than you did before. You got under the surface, and you didn't have to talk about ailments—what an older friend of mine calls 'an organ recital.'"

"Oh, that's good, that is, an organ recital! I want to remember that. I'm going to tell her that—some music!" We're laughing together.

She had made a few friends at the centre with common interests and they go to plays and concerts together. She had no time for that when she was working, but now she doesn't have to do as much planning. Her daughter says that she looks 60, not 74 and thinks her memory is all right—they have a few differences, and an argument can throw Rivka off a little bit from her "way of thinking rationally." But then she'll remember what a hard time her daughter had growing up without a father, and a mother working and tired all the time. And then they'll be all right.

"I'm glad to have a good relationship with both my daughters, but I'm careful about their sensitivities—like letting on I ever brought up children!"

"Or that you ever worked for a living!" We exchange the knowing looks of seasoned single parents.

"Mostly I don't forget like that, I remember because I do the dishwashing, and I know exactly where things are."

"So it's what you're used to."

"I'm a creature of habit," she replies, telling me how she organizes this week's theatre tickets in a little leather case, keys in a second compartment, cosmetics in another. She's not going to say, "I'll do it later," but has a place on a table in the hall, and whatever she wants to remember for the next day or so she puts there. That works unless she's rushing and forgets to look on the table. She laughs easily as she recalls one time when she went into her sister's room for something and left her little case on a chair and thought she'd left it wherever she'd been before and ran all over the place before she remembered she'd left it right in her room.

"Not in its customary place. I do that a lot. It's common for most people."

"I'm not putting it down to anything. I mean, some people, they're really scared, they think something has happened, that it has to do with aging, like a disease of aging in the brain. Like Alzheimer's."

"People are afraid of that, I know, but it wouldn't be the kind of forgetting you're describing."

"So what kind would it be?"

"If you forgot you kept your things in a little case."

Rivka looks happy. "Oh, I see, well, I'm a long way from forgetting like that!" And then she asks me if people became more forgetful as they age. We talk about factors that affect memory, such as illness, some kinds of medication or mixing medications, being poor, alone and isolated, which can have more impact than aging itself. "There are so many kinds of stress when you're old. One of the things that *is* different seems to be taking in new information a little more slowly as you get older, possibly because people take the time to think about things. Most older people will say that they need time for themselves."

"Oh, yes, definitely, if we didn't have it … I need that, I know I do."

"So, other than the things we've talked about, there is not much to say that aging is the cause of memory loss. You could put it the other way around and say that memory loss is the cause of aging …"

"Ha ha. Yeah, yeah, that's good, that is."

"… in healthy people. As we've said, physical illness can certainly be enough of a distraction …"

"… to slow you down," Rivka completes my sentence—"and when you slow down anywhere, it carries over, doesn't it?" And she asks me if a heart condition affects the brain. I reply that it depends on the condition, for instance if the carotid artery is blocked, then the brain doesn't receive enough oxygen—that's not aging, that's the condition, or it could be medication. Blood pressure pills can have an effect on memory, as well as on taste buds. Rivka looks satisfied, reporting that although her medication leaves an unpleasant taste, it doesn't worry her.

"So it sounds like …" I start to say.

"I'm getting better! Yes. I have a good memory. I feel better. I feel better within myself, and I feel healthier, despite the medication. Mentally I feel much better. Much better. My upbringing was Victorian—children should be seen and not heard at all. Upbringing does a lot. I mean, it doesn't affect everybody the same way."

"No, there are plenty of differences … and you're saying that now, where you have an area where you feel intimidated, you take that as an opportunity to do something about it, to work on that."

"Not to have a complex."

"So that you can work through that fear and not have it anymore, or at least it will be less than ..."

"That's right."

"And that's really improved how you feel about yourself."

"Exactly, yes. And yet we were laughing, my sister and I, she always says: 'Oh, you were always called the dolly' [the attractive child]. But it's a funny thing, I never thought about myself that way, there was too much of the other. But I think the biggest loss was my husband, because he was a loving and kind person, which I guess I needed."

"It sounds as if you didn't have such a loving and kind environment at home."

"No. No way."

"Hard-working parents, I suppose."

"Yes, yes."

"Who were just so busy that they didn't have time for much else."

"No, exactly."

"Did your mother work outside the home?"

"She was the regular one, worked all the time ... Dad, he worked when he felt like working. He was more of a scholar, and he had business reverses ... a very difficult person. However, that's all in the past."

Feeling that we are more comfortable together, I ignore the hint.

"Do you remember the past very well?"

"Oh, yes."

"How does it come back to you?"

"It comes through my sister a lot. She never married anyone, and she really got the bend of the stick. When we came here to Toronto, she was the one to stay with my parents when they got old. So every now and then, it flares up, and I say: 'I know, I know, but things are different now, you have me and my daughter, who is like your child you're so close, you go to concerts, you enjoy yourself—but I guess you can't help it once in a while. I've never got into it with the feelings of that story."

I see how that would cross the line for her and that not talking about the private/personal could be a family trait too—just as in my family. However, it serves as a springboard: "When you remember your past ... you know some people will smell something which reminds them, like the smell of fresh baked bread ..."

"Friday nights. The Sabbath was very important. We were scrubbed clean, you know. There was a little bit of baking, a little bit of buns and poppy seed cookies. And that was all. And I remember the harsh winters, living in small quarters 'cause things were really bad."

"Feeling ...?"

"Yes. Will we ever get out of this?"

"The sounds?"

"Of course. The chanting on Friday nights. My father had a good voice, but he was such a difficult man you couldn't appreciate those things."

"No pleasure in remembering those sounds."

"Absolutely not." She looks at me sideways, smiling a little, and then laughs ruefully, "I was not going to talk to you about that personally."

"No, you weren't, and we don't have to. Anything else about the past, not necessarily personal?"

She thinks for a moment and then refers to her education again: even in elementary school, it hadn't been "as good as it should have been. I missed two years of my life in grade school. I was passed on from grade two to four and then from six to eight. Now, I was no genius. I think they needed more space, and they didn't have enough desks in the classroom."

"What happened? Did that make you feel sort of ..."

"That was why I found high school very difficult, even grade eight was hard."

"I would think so!"

"Very hard. I don't know why they did it. Why did they do it? I was no genius, I know, I don't profess to be. But I was pretty good in grade two. Then in high school I had a little physics, I had chemistry, French, a little of this and that, you name it. But I didn't know what they were talking about."

The Heart of the Matter

I am moved by her poignant cri de coeur *and the way she goes to the heart of the matter.* "Those missed years made such a difference; you just didn't have the background. It was all too fast for you."

"Much too fast."

"Was there any plus side to it at all?"

"Well, I certainly learned how to concentrate, didn't I!"

"Well, you sure did! I'm always aware of how you keep us on track and how you look at someone straight on with your eyes and drink it all in. Like a sponge, it just goes in."

"It is a kind of protection—I mean, I had to be perfect—so alert, to get what I could. I don't like to think about it now, but I don't forget it." *(So like Miriam's childhood.)*

"No, I guess not, it's not something you would forget; it went on for a long time in the life of a child, in anyone's life for that matter."

There seems to be a mutual agreement not to go more deeply— after all, what more can she say now? As she might have put it, "That's it; it's over and done with."

And she asks what else is on the list from my memory workshop.

I invite her to select topics, and she picks "How you feel about what happened long ago" *(!)* and tells me that people touching her drive her wild. "Excepting my husband, I didn't mind, and I hug my daughter and kiss her every time she comes to dinner. But people have a habit of hugging me. Why do they *do* that? Someone said: 'Because they like you.' But I don't like it; you can have eye contact, talk to people that you're comfortable with."

"Some people are more physical than others and not too sensitive about those who aren't."

"I can't stand it when I even … you know, a friend of mine, she has long fingers, a nice person, but when she's talking to you, if you interrupt her, she'll put her hand on you, and I know she'd like to finish what she has to say."

"And that bothers you."

"It does, not that she wants to finish what she's saying but the way she does it, the touching. I mean, I don't show that I resent it, but some people do this"—holds my arm—"grab you, and I have to find a way to ease away. I don't know why I'm that way. I can't keep telling people, 'I can't stand when you touch me,' so my defence is that I've got arthritis …"—*long pause*—"… I was never abused as a child sexually, no, no, never."

"Maybe not touched enough, and so you're not used to it."

"Maybe not touched enough is more like it. Not enough hugs and kisses … I shrivel up … maybe not. And yet my sister who lives with me, she loves it, she'll go over to people and hug and kiss them. I can't do that."

"My sister's a big hugger too. She's only a year and a half younger, yet we're very different."

"I know I'm so different. I feel myself so different."

Her eyes are shiny, and I am close to tears … *and I know I must help us turn away from the pain of not being touched and grasp at the first thing that comes into my mind.*

"You know, the older we get," I continue, "the more different we become from one another."

"Within family and with other people?"

"Oh, yes, both ways. You know, it's easy enough to see the similarities in a group of 10-year-olds, even 18 and 25-year-olds, but the older we get, the more unlike each other we become."

We agree that this is because we develop our personalities. Rivka adds that her power of concentration has increased considerably.

"The past is very vivid for you."

"I can recall everything since four years old."

"And do you visualize those years, do you see a picture of them, as you described with …?"

"Oh, yes, I remember my aunt coming from the synagogue in very bitter cold in Winnipeg, and we had the Quebec heater, and she would sit there with her legs apart to get the heat coming to her whole body … and, oh my, my Dad, he … ha ha … that's pretty good, isn't it?"

Laughing with her, I say, "It sure is! What other sorts of things do you remember?"

"OK. Oh, listen, I've got to get home, you know the buses are very crowded."

We have become comfortable enough by now that I choose not to hear this as Rivka wanting to "walk away" from what we are talking about and offer to drive her home. With some reluctance she agrees, saying she has to see how her sister is doing, but can stay a little bit longer.

We continue to talk about other things she remembers, and she says, "Lifting all the heavy coats at the shop, I don't know, but my arms still ache, and my legs, because I was running up and down the stairs in the dress shop, lifting those heavy coats, dumping them on the hangers, helping the women—ladies in waiting! Huh! Obnoxious creatures! So, all that."

"Hurt your muscles."

"I guess it did."

"I guess they remember, don't they?"

"Pardon?"

"I guess they remember."

"My muscles … they remember … Yeah, they took it all in. Yeah. It's funny to think of it that way, I never have, but it's true isn't it, your muscles … your body … they have a way. Almost like they store things in there isn't it? Hmmm … They take it all in."

"Yes. They certainly do." *I don't pursue this, not wanting to spoil this moment.* I hold out the list—"Is there's anything we haven't covered?"

"I'm fine and dandy. About the pain in my lower back and leg problems, you know. I manage, I'm all right."

She is reassuring me! "You seem to be doing really well. I'm so glad, Rivka."

"We're just about finished, aren't we?"

"Yes, I think so, but just before we go I'd like to ask you—as long as you have the time—what you'd say to a group of young people about your experience of getting older and of your own memory—in spite of everything people hear about memory loss and aging."

"Well, do you think younger people have better memories than older people?"

"No, not really—when you take into consideration what we talked about a few moments ago, about all the situations that are big stressors for old people. Different ways of remembering maybe, and remembering different things, but not necessarily worse than younger people."

"Listening. That's a good way."

"And what have you found helpful as you've gone along your path that might help them someday?"

"Now that's a difficult question!"

"Is it?"

"Very difficult. Very, very difficult. It was difficult times, not even giving people the opportunity to think for themselves. So what can I say to younger people?"

"You've lived for 74 years, you've learned a lot during those difficult times."

"I've learned to relate to people, I've a lot more patience with them."

"And you've learned things that have helped you get to where you are now."

"Exactly."

"A lively, vital, intelligent person—So, if you were to give a young person some advice …?"

"Think positive. Think positive … And try to be patient and understanding and tolerant of people."

"And listen!"

"And listen, yes." We are both grinning, both of us getting the double meaning. "Keep on learning," she'd say to younger people, "but only if you want to." When she was young, "there was a certain pattern to life that all came down to economics, helping your parents pay the bills." Now she loves to learn new things, just for themselves, for the enjoyment, especially "new words, words that have colour to them ... I'm learning from you now."

"Really! What are you learning?"

"How to express myself ... like if I ask a question, you're filling in where I just sort of can't find a word, helping me find the words I want to use, a word that has a better way of imparting knowledge on a higher level, and that's what I aim for, a higher level all the time."

"I'm glad to hear that, because I think—well, you gave me the impression when I phoned that you were apprehensive about our getting together, maybe were having second thoughts."

"Well, I was—I guess I gave you a hard time, didn't I?" She looks at me as if she's wondering whether or not to smile and whether we can share this as a joke.

"Mmm, you did—but just a little. It didn't hold me back, though."

She laughs. "No, it didn't, did it! Well, I'm glad, now, that it didn't. You see, after I said I would, I thought it over, and I remembered a workshop I'd taken last year, and the lecturer didn't think much of what I told him about remembering intuitively, and that I knew where to go by landmarks and so forth."

"Maybe he didn't understand what a visual learner you are."

"Unnhh ... what do you mean?"

"Well, we talked about the way you learn kinaesthetically, through movement and your body. You've also talked about drawing a speech, words with colour, how you make pictures and visual associations of what to remember, that sort of thing. Do you recall the Roman Room exercise we did in class, how you can walk around a place and attach what you want to remember by visualizing a place—and you said you had fun with that, you already knew about it."

"Oh, yes—I condition myself that way—I do a lot of associations. You see, your mind tells you how to go about things so you know—more or less."

Simplifying

I ask Rivka whether she'd like a copy of the transcript of our conversation. No, she was at the age where she doesn't want more to look after, she was simplifying. "The easier to look after, the better." Now that she's not working, she just does the things that are important to her. She "feels her responsibilities" but just looks after the bare necessities—in order to let other stuff in.

"A certain amount of nurturing goes on for your sister."

"One hand washes the other, for sure. But I'm easier to get along with."

"Are you?"

"Yeah, I don't know whether it's because she had it worse at home. I don't see it, but I wonder—as you said, we're all different, even from the same family. But—ah—I do what I can."

"I know you do. I guess we should be going, so you can get back to her. It's been such a pleasure talking with you."

"I've enjoyed it. And you've been discrete. I thought I'd be very apprehensive, but it's all right."

"Oh, Rivka, thank you … and I think you've been very brave."

She reaches over and pats my hand, covers it with hers for a few moments. I give her hand a little squeeze, and then we stand up, put on our coats, and walk together to the parking lot.

Untold Stories

School like recess
from a lonely childhood,
left early for years of selling clothes
to picky women—I made my way,

married a loving man who died
too young to give our child
the tender girlhood I never had
and still yearn for.

Memories fade, new friends fill
the hollows, time opens for clay
in my hands words in my mouth,
long rambling walks,

music
surrounds me. Now, my tired arms
no longer ask
"Why did they do that?" I feel
myself so different—

my throat closes, forgetting
how it was.

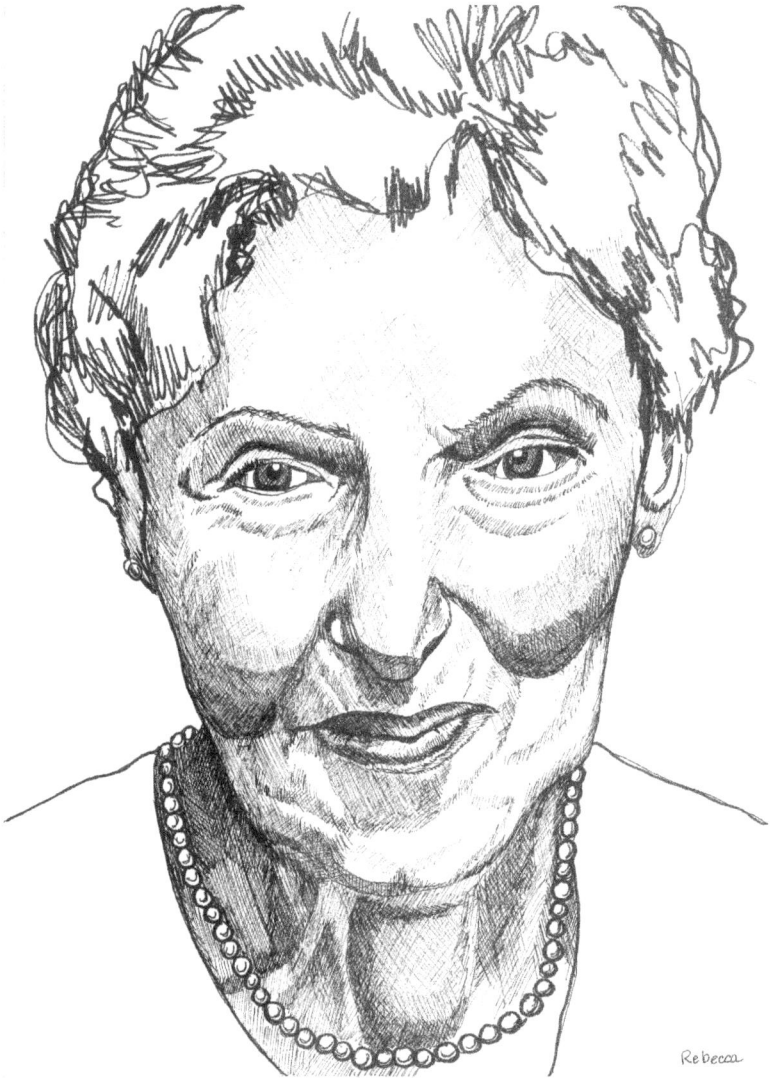

Rebecca

Standing Up: Rebecca's Story

"Stand up for yourself or you won't have any life at all."

A Closed Family

It's late fall and Rebecca wears an elegantly casual black coat, a touch of red in scarf and gloves. Almost black eyes and cropped, dark brown hair curling a little around aquiline features speak of Sephardic origins. We meet in the lounge of the seniors' centre where I had taught a course in memory strategies and she seems eager to get started. She'd been reading about some of the other people I had spoke with and after settling in with coffee Rebecca tells me that her parents might well have been one of the Portuguese herring eaters the child Emma saw in the steerage of the *Lake Ontario* as it sailed from Liverpool to Montreal. Her early life "was tough from the beginning." The second oldest in a European Jewish family of six—three daughters and three sons—she started taking care of her younger brothers when she was very young. She was 15 when the third one was born, and her mother, knowing that she was crazy about the kids, "gave him to me: 'Here,' she said, 'this one is yours.' To this day he feels like I am his Mom."

Every day was chores, school, more chores, and babysitting, and then homework when she had the time. "I had a zest for life, I still do. But I never had the chance to make as much of myself as I could have. My brothers had the chance; we worked to give it to them. My Dad was old school—men need an education. Maybe that was true, but my brain was as good as my brothers." She laughs. "I like to probe, teach myself, I always have. I read a lot of politics, can speak to anyone, don't feel I'm less educated than my doctor brother—I feel I know more about life than any of them. If you want to, you can learn anything. But the background I never had—the knowledge I should have had to get ahead when I was young—

I didn't have, because it's taken for granted you get married and don't need it." She did not marry.

At 19, weighing 90 pounds, she went to work in her brother-in-law's factory and quickly became forelady of 20 women workers. His sister-in-law was jealous of her promotion, wanted her position, and was given it. Rebecca was asked to help her with her new responsibilities, but she refused, telling her brother-in-law: "My ability is not going to be hers. At 19 (at that time 19 was a kid)—even at that time I had my nerve, was outspoken. I'm not that dumb." The business started to go downhill, the other women "were laughing," so Rebecca became manager again and stayed for two years. "If I'd helped her she'd still be forelady, and I'd still be sitting down sewing, and running around for her. But I didn't feel good. I was underpaid and unhappy in a dead-end job. That's why I left. And I was ruining my life living at home. I still had a lot of responsibilities there, and my mother was jealous because at 15 Sam was like my own. I looked at myself, said: 'The whole thing is no good. I'm getting lost in this shuffle.'"

Her older sister, who had refused to look after her brothers, had married, had moved to Detroit, and had two boys of her own. She asked Rebecca to come and help out while her husband was away during the war. Rebecca went. Her mother "wrung my heart, telling me how much Sam missed me, to get me back. My poor mother, she had no help once I was gone. She said Sam wanted to visit—she thought once I saw him I'd change my mind. But I said: 'No, you don't. He's OK' (and he was, he was growing up). We had to break the ties. It took 10 years, but we got away from it … It was hard. I couldn't know then, but it turned out to be a good move for me."

She and her sister's two little boys were crazy about each other, but she soon realized that she was becoming too involved in their life, just as she had with her brother's at home. She knew it wasn't good for her, she was going to get stuck there and make herself sick again. Although she felt terrible, and knew her sister would miss her help, she moved to New York to lead more of her own life.

Rebecca enjoyed her life in New York but used to be so anxious to see the children that she'd go on the weekend to Detroit. "To this day, the boys are just like mine, but I had to let go of that too. I cared inwardly, but that was their life I was in. I was living their life, not my own. Especially when you're single, you have to learn to stand up for yourself, for your rights or you won't have any life at all and you go downhill."

"And feel bad?"

"Yeah, not well at all."

"Those years gave you some wonderful memories though?"

"Oh yeah, they're like my children. But I don't dwell on it—you can't. When I take things as they come, I'm better."

A Room of Her Own

After leaving Detroit, she did piecework in a millinery factory in New York for several years. The pay was bad, and she was so tired that she "couldn't spend what I had." As well, her health was deteriorating again, so she left for a much better job selling hats at Peck and Peck, eventually becoming manager of the department. "From then on, no one bothered me, and life was easier."

"You supervised the staff. Did you do some of the buying as well?"

"Oh, yes, most of it. I knew my customers."

"One of my mother's sisters went to New York to learn the garment trade," I said. "She must have been there about the same time as you were. That was pretty daring in those days, wasn't it, for a woman to go to a big city on her own?"

"Yes, it was. I didn't have a lot of approval. But I had some good times."

"Many memories."

"Oh, yes," she laughs softly. "With my sister's children, when they got old enough to visit, showing them around. And on my own. I went out with a lot of men, some wanted to marry me, but it was my choice not to marry." *(I couldn't help wondering about Aunt D.'s life in New York and hoping she had a good time, too! All I knew was that she came home qualified to teach "domestic science" in high schools, and never married.)* To remember the good times, Rebecca imagines them; to coax herself out of an unhappy mood, she tries not to think about the bad times, she pushes them away, or they get her down in the dumps.

"So, sometimes it's not so easy to forget," I say. "Seems to be unhappy things that people don't forget. What do you think?"

"Yeah, because it's deeper—don't you think?"

"Some people seem to be able to block out horrifying events—like some of the people I've met in Dr. F.'s holocaust survivors groups. He was one himself, you know."

"Yes, well, they don't, really. They never forget. When you revive it every year, it's terrible. I knew a couple, she was only 15, she goes into remission after these meetings, she's ill for months. Too much reliving for her. Once it's deep you never forget, no matter what people say. Forgive maybe, that's hard enough, if you can. But forget? Never. It's your life, how can you forget that?"

"The deep ones are always there, then. What *can* you forget?"

Forgetting—and Remembering

Rebecca says that for the sake of family relationships it's important to try to forget the injustices done to you in your family. Like Meyer, she thinks that if you make an effort not to dwell on them, to forgive and move on with your own life, in time they don't seem so important, which makes it easier to remember the good times. She wants to remember what has meant a lot to her—and, although she'd like them to be, the meaningful times weren't always the happy ones. I ask her what she thinks someone means if they tell her they have a "good memory."

"That their life was good—that's a good memory. About someone you loved, your family."

"How about a memory that functions well?"

"I imagine they had a good life, don't you think so?"

"An easy life ... and so easy to remember?"

(I am not sure yet how she uses the words "good," "bad," " memory," or "easy," for that matter. Easy how? Where?)

"Yes, the bad experiences—what most people have—if you have a little bit of brains ... you think more ..."

"And when you think more?"

"Gives you a better insight on life ... doesn't it?" Long pause. "I didn't have such a good life."

"No?"

"No. But I try to make it what I can. I think about the good things, and I'm grateful for what I have—but it makes me feel sad to talk about it ... Talking brings it out."

Long pause. Her feelings about the dark parts of her life evoke mine about mine.

"In a long life—it's not so joyous ... sometimes hard to avoid that," I say.

Rebecca is crying now, and I am too—*(it's hard to keep on forgetting the not-joys of my own life)*. I rummage in my purse for tissues for us both, and then she says, trying to laugh a little:

"Isn't this ridiculous!"

And I try to match her joking tone: "What have you got against tears?"

"It's self-pity."

"Well, then, I am full of self-pity, because I often feel sad."

"Yeah? This is good, though. I don't have people here I can talk to."

"Tears don't bother me."

"No?"

"Not at all."

She laughs, relieved. "Oh!"

"I am honoured that you share your feelings with me."

"I have a feeling towards you, too." She puts her hand out, and we hold hands as we talk. "Why I think I'm sad. My sister lost her husband eight years ago, and now she's sick, and that bothers me."

"Of course, it does. The one you lived with?" Rebecca nodded. "Oh, then you're close to her. What's the matter with her?"

"A heart attack. She's fine ... but since he left ... he was the strong one, and now ..."

"Is she coming here?"

"Oh, no, we couldn't live together. We don't get along too good in our ideas. I could have helped her, but she wouldn't let me. She got it from stress, and I could see ... When I used to talk to her: 'I don't want to hear it,' she'd say. I gave her a lot of literature to read—those writers must have recognized her!—but she didn't want it, never used to listen to me. And now, she wants me to go to her. It bothers me that she's alone. She has a daughter who's good to her, but since she's sick, I feel terrible."

"You're really struggling."

"Yes. We're different types. I couldn't live with her, but I love her. I spoke to her on Friday, and she said: 'Well, you gotta learn to live with it.' Well sure, I've had to learn to live with what I've got. But she thinks I've had it easy. She's had a good life—even though she's sick now, her memory is still good."

I told her that I have a younger sister whom I love dearly, but that we can't live together for more than a couple of days. "We both try ... It's sad, not much to do about it, we're very different people, but it is sad."

"Everybody has something," Rebecca agrees.

She will go to her sister, just as she did to help her out when her husband was away fighting in the war and for those seven years when their mother was sick. Back then, "being away that long put a real crimp in my career, I can tell you, but I was the unmarried one. The boys were good sons, but she had no daughters nearby." Now Rebecca is free to stay as long as she wants to, but three months "is as long as I can stand it." There will be another friend with them for a while, which will make it easier, but she's not looking forward to just sitting around doing nothing or going to malls. "I'm doing it for her. You do for your family."

A Full Life

She never made much money, but at 62 Rebecca had saved enough to quit her job while she was still young enough to enjoy living in New York and do all the things she didn't have time for while she was working. She "really lived" and had her "fill of lectures, concerts, plays and art galleries, nice dinners, and trips here and there," and then, when she turned 70, she moved back to Toronto, where her brothers and their families live. She knows that as she ages she cannot be alone. To be alone and not to be able to tell your story is "to forget your life." And you "have to have someone in back of you." She was sad to leave her good friends in New York and the life she had, "but friends cannot look after you when you are sick. I have a good family."

Now that she is retired, she finds that it's wonderful not to have to get up—she has "been standing up for a long time." There has been so much turmoil in her life; now she can slow down and take it easy. She manages, has no children to leave money to, is not a big spender, has her nest egg put by. She is able to get everything together and relax: "I'm more at ease with myself, at peace you might say. I still love it, every day to do what I want."

"Sounds like a good place to be ..."

"Yup. My brother's kids, they love me too, they made a party and gave me two chi for my birthday. Do I look 70?"

"No, you don't."

"Everybody says. I think it's because of my sense of humour. Also, I like to teach myself, to learn something new—I came to your memory workshop because I like to be involved with people and learning."

She tells me that she actively makes her memory work for her and has already used many of the techniques from the workshop, especially the exercises on stress and the sensory organizational methods such as imagery and association.

Rebecca doesn't worry about her memory. She thinks some forgetting can't be helped, but it's sad when people forget and have no memories about their lives. And she thinks it's just as bad to be sick, inactive, and live only in the past. Like her uncle who was a union member and didn't like her brother-in-law any better than she did.

"He's [her uncle] not so young. Kinda sad, the way he is now, nothing to look forward to; it's all in the past." Thinking about Avram, another member in the workshop, I ask her if he feels good when he talks about his working days, has no trouble remembering them.

"No, but now—he hasn't made a life."

Some of the workshop members had planned to meet now that classes had finished, and I ask Rebecca if she is joining them. She's quick to say that she had enjoyed the class but the group is not for her. "Lovely people, but too old in their attitude." She says she can still learn anything she wants to and that her memory "is as good as it was 30 years ago, not much difference with age."

She thinks that older people forget names and dates and appointments because of illness, or their life situation—being poor "makes you forget everything else," and being alone too much is "a recipe for disaster"; no one cares, so there is no point in remembering. "Otherwise, for a good memory, maybe they never had a good memory in the first place." She can remember when she was five, which impresses her sister, whose daughter says her mother doesn't want to remember. Rebecca understands this—"with the life we had"—but this isn't forgetting, it's just not dwelling on the things you'd rather not think about.

She thinks she is still interested in learning and has no trouble with her memory because she keeps herself young by looking after her health, making sure she exercises, doesn't harbour the past so she can get enough sleep, and eats a correct diet. Diet is especially important, since she developed diabetes 20 years ago. If she doesn't pay attention to her "red-light" foods, she can feel dizzy and ill, and then she "can draw a blank. As I said, when you're not feeling well, you can forget. I live accordingly, I use my common sense—you learn how to handle it. In the beginning it was tough, though."

I tell her a little about my experiences with hypoglycaemia, how it affects my concentration, memory, and general sense of well-being, and that I find it hard to stick to a rigid diet. Like me, she said that she feels sleepy when she strays off the path, but "that's not age, it can happen to anyone. Children can have insulin problems, too—but there are diseases of old age that can affect the mind, aren't there?"

"Well," I reply, "the older we get, our whole body slows down, including our immune system, so more can happen—bones, digestion, that sort of thing—distractions that can affect your concentration, your attention."

"But if you look after yourself, you can slow that down too—I've read about that."

"Sure you can. And you learn how to manage slowing down, giving yourself time. As you do."

"I do my best. I remember a lot of things. Once in a while I forget, but I'm pretty alert."

Being involved with interesting people who are upbeat and still learning is important to her, because she finds it harder to forget the bad times when she is alone, and they can take over. This is not good, because she wants to have a good memory. As well, if she lets herself go, she can start forgetting other things, and when she forgets "like that," it upsets her.

"What do you mean by forgetting 'like that'?"

"What I've been reading, or what I learned in a lecture. Things like appointments and so forth don't bother me especially. I put them in a book."

"Yeah, that's what I do. I say to people that I have to write it down, that part of my mind is in that book."

"Well, you can't remember everything. But if I start forgetting what I've learned, like in a conversation, it's distressing. I feel as if I'm not all there."

"As if part of you is missing?"

"Yeah, it is, don't you think so? When my memory is good, I feel more alive."

"Which memory?"

"Any memory. Another thing I regret is not having an education. Oh, I wish I had. You see? It comes back, those feelings keep coming back."

Rebecca's Dilemma

At this point in our conversation I think that in a way Rebecca is living a paradox. Forgiving her family for the early life she had, and the choices made for her that she would never have made for herself, has become part of her daily meditation— which means trying to forget: forgetting the unhappy parts of her life and remembering only the good ones, so she could feel alive. But to keep on learning and remembering as much as she could whenever she had the chance, and not to forget what she had learned, she has to focus on remembering, not forgetting, and that keeps her active—and alive. She has to remember and forget almost at the same time, and that seems contradictory.

But the contradiction is in my mind, not hers. I have been confused by what she means by a good and a bad memory, until I realize she is using the same words to describe two different kinds of memory, each of which she experiences in both cognitive and sensory ways.

It is clear that, for Rebecca, having a good memory means having had a good life, and having a bad memory refers to the parts of her life that had been unhappy. At first, I thought she was referring to specifically good and bad memories that she remembered with pleasure or pain. But she wasn't, she was talking about a state of well-being or ill-being, about feeling good, or unwell and distressed emotionally and/or physically.

Having a good memory means feeling physically and emotionally well, feeling alive, being more at peace with herself, so that she can take things as they come and accept that she made her life and that it's been good overall. A bad memory is about things that are deeper and hard to forget, when she feels sick and cannot "pull herself up," or when she is sad—"down in the dumps, in a funny mood, sad and disappointed" in her life.

Rebecca doesn't talk about remembering names or dates or appointments as good or bad; she uses common strategies such as lists or a daily diary. Or she can "call them up" by not worrying and taking the time to think or visualize. Because the other kind of good or bad memory that concerns her is the memory that allows her to remember information, to be able to "probe, to teach" herself. To make up for her lifelong regret about not having had the education that would have given her a better life, she determined to be a lifelong learner. Any threat to that is enough to make her feel sick all over.

To live with this tension, she had to learn that it was all right to care for herself, as well as for other people. She "works on forgiveness," and it's still important for her to care for other people—to keep connected. But she tries to make looking after herself a priority. This is one of the hardest lessons she has ever had to learn—and, as she observes, she is still learning how to do this, as well as how to keep on accepting herself as a self-caring person, a person with "rights."

"It may look as if I've been selfish because I'm alone, but I never used to care too much for myself, just for others, until, like I said, I decided I had to care for myself."

"Made a big difference in your life?"

"Oh, yes. Now that I can think of myself, I feel better, I look after myself better. I had to push the children away. I can say no, which I never used to. I still care a lot, but I had to learn to stand up for my rights, for myself."

"Sounds like you have."

"Especially when you're single."

I share with her my some of my experiences about being single and comment that learning to give myself permission to look after myself was not a one-time decision for me but "seems to go on for a long time."

"Oh, it still is, don't you think?"

We say together, laughing: "It never stops!"

"You've been a really independent person," I say.

"Very much. Took a long time. I like it now; I'm as good as anybody else. I'm no better. This is the way to live."

"While you've had a hard life, you seem to be saying that you feel OK about yourself and the choices you made, about living independently and not being married. You know you did the right thing."

"Oh, yes, I even sent money when they needed it."

"You did the right thing for you?"

"For me? No."

"No? What would you have done differently?"

"Married. Had my own life."

"But you have been saying that you *have* had your own life."

"Life like it should be. Marriage. I'm not sorry, but I should have."

"What should you have …?"

"Children, I suppose."

"Well, in a sense you've had children, you've always been very involved with your nieces and nephews …"

"I might have married the wrong guy, and things wouldn't have been right—I talk that way, you know."

"To remind yourself that you had good reasons?"

"Yeah," she laughs, "that's it."

"That the way you grew up, you stayed away from marriage … Now, as you look back, you wonder if it wouldn't have been better to have had your own children … to look after you?"

"Nobody has to look after me. I'm clear. No one ever gave me. I gave them."

"So what would have been the advantage?"

"You know, the Jewish religion, to the community it's the wrong choice—if you're not married, it's shameful ... not to have children ... to carry on."

"You feel embarrassed?"

"No, not any more. I never did. Why should I? I know it's my own choice. I had a lot of men that wanted me. I guess I was afraid. When I saw someone getting serious I got rid of them. To me, marriage, what I saw, it was a lot of grief and strife. I'm not sorry about that, but ..."

"Not the right choice in your community, but the right choice for you, and it's been hard living it."

"Mmm. Yes, it has."

I tell her about some of the experiences of my three unmarried aunts—about her age—and what they thought about marriage, having children when there was no reliable method of birth control and the physical and emotional toll it takes, finishing with one of them telling me that she hadn't died of a heart attack, as my mother had, because she never married and had children.

"You know, that's true, it's really true."

"She said: 'I can look after myself.'"

"Like me."

"Very much like you. She's had her problems, like everyone else, but she's always been able to look after her health."

"I can see it from my brother's and sister's children. There's a lot of grief, a lot of grief—and my sister is sick."

A Lasting Regret

Rebecca went on to comment that, even though marriage and children would have meant a better life in the eyes of the Jewish community, she still would never have had the education she always longed for. This is her biggest regret, the one that is so hard to let go. "I could have used more education. I would have had some background, been more outgoing, had a better career." She would like to have studied medicine, like her brother. Although he is a nice fellow, he complains about not having had the money to become a specialist, "does not realize how lucky he is to be a doctor. And my sister who married this wonderful man, educated, an attorney, he nearly broke my heart—he was so kind, like a brother—when he died—Oh … But she had a good life."

"You don't think you've had a good life?"

"Yeah, in a way. I gave it to myself. I think I did."

"Sounds to me like you did."

"I've been around, I've seen things, have a nest egg put away so I don't have to go to anyone—I made sure I had that before I started to live—No. Not bad. Could have been better but …" Laughs. "I don't regret not being married, I regret not being educated."

We talked about what she has learned as she has lived her life, is still learning, and that professional people are often not educated in that sense. I mention that if she wanted something more formal, there's Elderhostel and University of the Third Age.

Rebecca replies that it's too late for her, now that she's older. And besides she worries that she won't be able to get the right diet. We talked about this for a while—managing diets and living away from the comforts of home—and then she spoke about not wanting to be with sick old people who have the wrong attitude. Like the ones she had met at the workshop—these people scare her and make her sad, not just because they are forgetful in the usual way, but because they remind her of the parts of her life that make her feel unhappy or sick and "give her a bad memory."

I tell her about my mother's friend Beatrice, whose injuries from a car accident were so serious that she had to move to a seniors' residence. Despite being in a home—which she never wanted—and being disabled and in pain a lot of the time, she is still going to as many of the adult education seminars as she can: the accommodations are quite comfortable and the staff have to pay attention to people's diets—so many with special needs.

"Like you, it's important for her to be with people still keen to learn. The residents in the home don't seem to be. There are so few people she can talk to there—mostly the staff and they don't have a lot of time to talk with the residents."

Rebecca looks at me quizzically—perhaps thinking that I am trying to talk her into something?—and then asks: "This education, is it in the summer?" As I tell her more about the variety of programs—everything from history and astronomy to the arts—her eyes brighten, and she looks thoughtful. "Well, it wasn't so bad, my life, I don't dwell on the bad parts so much; I forget, I have to. I had a lot of laughs … and I have a good memory."

"You've learned a lot from your life that has made you …"

"What I am! Me."

"… and that you made a good life for yourself. And for other people too. You made a difference in other people's lives, not just your own: your family, friends, your colleagues. And you learned from them too."

"Yes, I did."

"In a sense you forget, in a sense …"

"It's there."

"You created the life you wanted?"

"Yes, I did. You take what you get and learn to live with it, and that's life. It's been OK."

Leave-taking

I walk away, I do not stay to see the eyes
pulling me back
— although I can feel them in the centre of my
shoulder blades—
waiting, not understanding

that leave-taking is not disowning, is not
forgetting or failure or sickness or not caring.

I need a lot of distance to figure out
how to remake connections later.
To see how the pattern is repeating
this time.

Some pasts never get older, and
there are some to which we can never return.
I cannot go back to a time when it wasn't there,
to a mind that doesn't keep running into
"Is there any returning ever?"

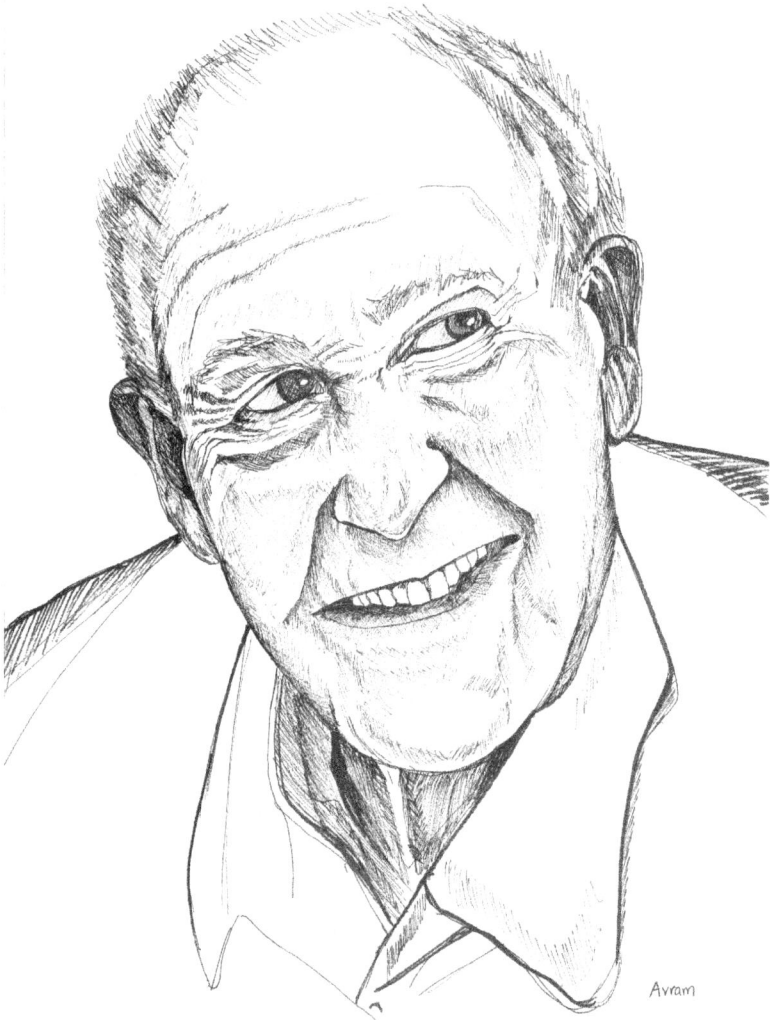

Avram

A Union Organizer Retools: Avram's Story

"Your life can seem over when you retire."

Avram is talking as he opens the door, saying how sorry he is to have forgotten our appointment. I reassure him as we walk down the hall to the living room talking, and then he laughs—embarrassed he hasn't taken my coat. Urging me to sit down, he tells me his wife is looking after the grandchildren but has left the tea things all ready. And he hurries out to put on the kettle.

I can see him from the pass-through—short, trim, brown hair just beginning to grey, broad forehead creased. While he moves around the kitchen, his stiffness speaks his worry. As he takes out milk and puts cookies on a plate, I ask him what he thought about the workshop on memory strategies at the seniors' centre a few weeks earlier. It was good, he'd liked it: "The only problem with me is, when you called, I knew there was a date missing, but for the life of me I couldn't connect it. I thought and I thought, but the thought never entered my head it was about the course, and I began to recollect and recollect and I said, 'How the hell could I have missed it?' You see, I usually mark it down. I have a pad, and I have a corkboard, I leave myself messages, and when I went and looked there was nothing. Nothing there."

It was different when he was working. His union jobs—first in Montreal, then the war years, and afterwards Toronto—took him all over Ontario and Quebec troubleshooting, and he had to be on his toes. He'd meet people and think to himself, "'OK, what's the name, where did I see them, what were we doing?' I didn't have any trouble remembering then."

"Because once you found the place, or what happened, the name came?" I ask.

"Oh yes. Because then, when I met them, I knew who they were. Before the meeting started someone would come over with a problem—there's always a problem, whether it's serious or not—and you'd talk. I never had to grope for that, like I do now."

"How is it different now?"

"Maybe because it's not the same kind of activity; no activity at all, really."

Montreal: Early Days

The son of Russian Jews, Avram was born and brought up in Montreal and lived and worked among francophones. In the late 1920s, at 16, he was apprenticed to the millinery trade. He joined the Hatters' Union, one of the country's oldest, founded in the 1870s, and rose from union head in Montreal to provincial and then national representative, liaising with all the associated unions. Avram told me about the early days of the labour/socialist movement in Quebec, Ontario, and the northern United States, colourful, action-oriented stories flowing effortlessly one after another: "You had to be sort of a half-baked diplomat. You had to divide your thinking you know, between the position of the employer, for the sake of the job, and the coconuts we had in the union to protect them from the vultures. There was no such thing as peace of mind. I had no vacations."

He learned to get as much as he could for workers without risking their jobs—although sometimes it could be close. For example, having been a labourer, Avram liked any technology that helped workers: they were "people, not tools; their problems were big for them." And so he would try to show management that "any problem with a worker is a problem for the company." He'd seen the latest machines in New York's millinery factories and advised the John B. Stetson Co. in Montreal to invest in them. But "those Englishmen" didn't see it that way. They looked down on the workers and their representatives, and everyone else for that matter, and kept putting him off. He tired of it.

"I didn't come in with the attitude of 'I have to submit,' and told them: 'Now look you people, you're using outdated machines here, you got a big name, you should have the latest.' 'Uh no, not for them,' they said, so I talked to my president, and I says, 'You know, those coconuts down there, they're stupid, they don't realize it's money for them, and better for the workers—for whom they couldn't care less—so anyway what we are prepared to do is to lend them the money to buy the new machines.'"

The company rebuffed him. "Who did they think was doing the work?" Avram "gave the boys the signal, 'cause I don't want anybody to salute to the bloody high command. I told them they got an obligation to do their job, but no extra duties—they don't appreciate them anyway."

They worked to rule for about six months. Management could do nothing because they followed all the rules, and the workers held fast because they knew Avram couldn't, and wouldn't, cave in. Finally the company gave up and sold out to become a branch of a big manufacturer in Philadelphia. Their attitude, Avram tells me, was to iron out the problem, not stand on a high horse in the way of progress.

In the Thick of the Action

Avram recalls the union activities readily and in detail. When I ask him why, he replies that what has happened a week ago is the same as this week or the week before and hard to recall.

"Nothing that hooks your interest?"

"Uh-huh, but when I was working I was in the middle of things, back and forth with everyone, having to keep track of a hundred things."

He picks up the story, remembering how the new American owner used to say to him, "Well Avram, this guy is Jewish, you handle him." "Ninety per cent of the factories in Quebec and Ontario were Jewish-owned. And some would only stoop—forgive my language—they were bastards, real bastards. They used to try to take advantage of the wage rates, especially with immigrants who didn't know ... they robbed the workers by not paying them the proper rate."

I mention that Rebecca, from the same memory workshop, had told me how her brother-in-law would not pay her the same wage as the men and refused to promote her. She decided to leave before they fired her for "being too demanding."

"They'd label her a whistleblower," Avram says. "She wouldn't get to first base." He tells me that hers was a common situation before unions and that, even with a union, employers would try to cheat workers whenever they could. He used different strategies, depending on the situation. For instance, he could demand to see the books—if they refused he could call a strike. "So they'd either give us the books or pay the proper rate."

He had other methods, too, and gleefully recalls them "as if they were yesterday." Like when the union saw that management was breaking the contract. The union was supposed to report to the labour board, but it might take three months to respond. "We'd say, 'Well look, Mr. __, we'll tell you what we'll do, we'll have to shift him over to another job.' Once that happened, four or five other workers started to shift over, a manoeuvre to show them we wouldn't let them get away with it." Many times owners would work after hours to save on overtime, knowing they were breaking the law, so the union would take them to court: "The law is the law, and it's better we had control of the situation."

He developed good relations with people who had climbed to middle management and were willing to "smooth the way." "I remember this one guy. He used to be a carpenter, then he was a foreman. He used to tip me off about what was happening on the floor so we could catch a situation before it got blown up. Then the manager, he'd say to me, 'Avram, what are you, a magician?' And then he'd give me another problem: 'Avram, I can't get this nutball to do anything, use your

discretion on that, will you? He bugs me day in and day out.' …
You had to be a psychiatrist sometimes to know where they
were coming from."

"Learning about people's personalities and quirks, how
to fit them all together and…"

"You bet. Drove me almost crazy myself at times, but
mostly I loved the challenge."

Anglo-French Relations

The Anglo owners couldn't seem to grasp that the millinery
trade was different in Ontario and Quebec, as were labour-
management problems and tactics. "They thought, because
they ran a factory, they knew everything. But *the workers knew the
people wearing the hats.* They could tell them, if they'd listen. But
they wouldn't." Avram listened, "training my mind to
remember."

He was systems manager for the union and knew that
the francophones did not know much English. So he would
speak French in union meetings and the workers would
applaud him. Sometimes he'd get stuck and ask "*S'il vous plaît,
expliquez. J'oubliez le mot.*" Everyone helped. The anglophone
officers wouldn't learn French or even have an interpreter.
"They had the attitude we were nobodies, and I didn't like
that."

They were so ignorant about French-Canadian culture
and society that he would try to fill them in, telling them that
the French had arrived long before the English and "were
entitled to all those churches and stores." But there was a big
divide between the well off and the workers and their families,
who were poor and didn't speak English. "So we went ahead
and established an English course for them. In Montreal we
had something like 600 members; 100 of them at a time took
advantage of those classes."

He understood the workers' situation and stood up for
them even in the most difficult circumstances: "Like when
some of the coconuts we had in the union, some of them

would come in half tanked. Another group we had, all of them were drunk all the time, absolutely drunk. And I'd get a call, 'Avram, come down here, we got a problem with this guy Jones.' Now I come down and I tell him, 'My goodness anyway, don't forget Jones has six kids, and his wife, poor thing, skinny as a rake and always in a turmoil with him, with his drinking.' I remember I told him I'd go to the (Canadian) president, have a talk about how the guy couldn't pay the rent. They paid the rent."

War Years

As he refills the teapot and replenishes the cookie plate Avram tells me how much he enjoys talking about the old days and asks me if anyone in my family had served in the Second World War. I told him about my uncle, who was a chaplain with the air force, and an aunt who was in the army. Avram said that he was exempted from military service because they needed people with his union experience and negotiating skills to handle the tough wartime labour situation. He remembers being embarrassed; some people thought it was because "he was a Jew he got let off."

Like Lev and some of the others I talked to, once Avram has a "key" word or image the scene unrolls before him in all its sensory detail and I feel as if I am right there with him as he picks up on another wartime image, remembering how he also helped European refugees, most of them Polish, before, during, and after the war. As the representative of both the union and the Trade and Labour Council he would meet with Catholic and Protestant clergymen to find jobs, homes, and clothes for the people they sponsored. He recalls how "the Jewish people were overabundant with donations. But when it came to honest-to-goodness relationships with any of the refugees, it wasn't there. Catholic or Protestant, whatever country they'd come from, they were immigrants and never in the same position as the wartime refugees. It was mostly the people who had been poor peasants in their own country before they came here who understood the need for clothes and food. But they had a . . . well you see they didn't want to get close. I think maybe they didn't want to go back there and those people took them back, you know."

"You mean they didn't want to remember?" I ask.

"No, they didn't. There are plenty of things people don't want to remember. Like I don't like to think about the way the Jewish factory owners treated immigrants. I must admit that my Jewish element showed poor respect for their neighbour, and I put my foot down on it. Someone would come in and they would be Anglo-Saxon and the owner would start talking to me in Yiddish. Well, as a courtesy to the individual you don't do that. You talk in English. The Jews tell me they express themselves better. Well, if we do that to our own it's a different ball game. You know a lot of those Jews came from Poland, and I don't know what the hell, Poland must have been a hellhole. Those Jews had mean tendencies. They didn't try to understand the other side of the story. You see once you weren't Jewish you weren't kosher. They'd say, 'That's a goy,' which means you're dumb."

"And you don't matter?"

"Yeah, that's it. But I wouldn't let them do that."

Avram's negotiating skills were invaluable in dealing with the Department of Immigration, which wouldn't accept refugees unless sponsors could guarantee them jobs. But, as Avram says, the refugees could clearly not take a job immediately, and he would have to get that through to officials. He did that by asking *them* to remember that they'd been immigrants once themselves, maybe not refugees, but they did know what it was like not to speak the language "or to be so hungry you couldn't think." *I can see them being pulled in as Avram connected them to images of their own lives, even ones they wanted to forget.* Once again the union sponsored classes and installed extra machines to give the newcomers practice working on them.

Union-Management Politics

There *were* quite a few communists in the Hatters' Union. Avram's boss, Manny, would often receive letters from company managers accusing Avram of being a left-winger. Avram chuckles: Manny would call him in and ask him what he knew. Avram would explain it to him. Manny would ask, "Is that all?" And Avram would reply, "'Yeah, that's all,' and he'd accept it. We went through quite a few trials and tribulations. We had to buck the National Catholic Syndicate as well ... You see I was a peacemaker. And we had a lot of left-wingers. In fact we controlled the thing if we wanted to."

"Peacemakers were called left-wingers in those days? They were the socialists, weren't they?"

"Yes, exactly, the socialists. It's the same today."

"Like, for example, the French Canadians being under the influence of the Catholic church," Avram explains. "They were told time and time again—which we didn't know until we were told about it by some of the French-Canadian members—that they had no rights. They relied on us to be more aggressive. Whenever there was a strike they used to come over to our union. You see we were very active. We had a perfect reputation in that sense."

The membership was young, lively, and forging a new kind of labour movement. The "old hands"—for them, "everything was ... Trade and Labour Council"—opposed the younger members, who were more attuned to worker's rights, and they had some fierce battles.

Avram was firm. "Our union didn't care if we were dictatorial. We knew we were on the right track for the workers. But the thing was I had the patience to talk to them. Possibly the others didn't know how to cope with the problem so they'd just let it ride or whatever."

"That was your job, talking to so many different kinds of people all the time—you really perfected those skills."

"Well yes, I did. With negotiations, your attitude was so important. You had to understand the background of both sides, not just the immediate problem."

This meant that he was "here, there, and everywhere," as he says, juggling the workplace and wage needs of workers and the demands of owners, managers, and foremen, while trying "to fit everything in with all the rules and regulations they made to try and make some sense for both sides."

I remark that he must have used every memory strategy and negotiating trick in the book—had probably invented a few of his own. He replies that he had to, and that was part of what he loved about his job. But it was stressful, because the demands were continuous and "being in an oppositional position a lot of the time didn't help."

Organizing in Toronto

After the war Manny asked Avram to take on a job in Toronto where the people who had taken over the local were encountering so many problems that nothing they did seemed to work. "You understand how to talk to these people, Avram. I'm asking you to take it on, be the manager."

Avram went, but he never had a quiet moment. He found that the local's executive board had very little respect for French Canadians in Ontario. It couldn't understand them. And so it ignored or, worse still, couldn't even see the ways the anglophone foremen and workers discriminated against them. "They looked down on us as if we were back in the woods, like we were Indians or something (no disrespect intended). So, needless to say this wasn't appreciated."

He would have to explain to them that when a French-speaking member doesn't understand English it's their responsibility to try to explain to them. They got nowhere with them, so once again Avram had to get tough: "'Now look, if we have any discriminatory tactics, it's not the French speakers being difficult or causing problems, it's the English speakers, Jews, Gentiles, whoever, that are the problem, and we're not going to tolerate it. Now the next member, worker or foreman, who steps out of line is going to be penalized a week's pay, board or no board.'"

Nevertheless, he could not convince the executive to accept his way of negotiating, of interacting with both sides until they reached an agreement. And then, when he had to "lay down the law" about drunkenness, the union too gave him such a hard time that he felt he "wasn't getting anywhere with anybody." He knew the workers were poor and struggling and resented their treatment. Avram hated it too, but he also knew that drunkenness would simply make things worse.

"It was almost impossible to get them to see that. They didn't see any change with the management you see, or even their own union executive. You could hardly blame them."

"You put up with an awful lot, didn't you?" I prodded. "From both sides. And you were away from home, in unfamiliar territory, and without the kind of support you had in Montreal."

"It was pretty bad. It's amazing. You know, I said it before, but it's true, there was so much, you had to be a psychiatrist to understand."

"To see everyone's point of view and then get them to understand each other."

"Yeah, like that. It takes its toll too. **A**fter six years, I was on the verge of colitis. The doctor told me, 'Avram, you can't stay in this job too long because I can't help you. You don't know how to rest.'" Avram observes: "I loved that job; it just got to be too much for me."

After the Union

After he left union work in Toronto, Avram had several jobs and then started his own business making and selling novelties. He'd always loved football, had played in Montreal with both intermediate and senior teams, and watched every game at the Canadian National Exhibition stadium in Toronto. At one game he met a former teammate who introduced him to the people who operated tourist stands. They started to buy his novelties because they were cheaper and better quality than the ones from the United States. Business was very good for a number of years, then fell off, and he sold the operation.

What did he do now? "Not enough. [In] retirement I don't do anything much. This is the problem. I get up in the morning, look at the news. There's nobody. Nothing here, so I have to get out. I run down to the Exhibition, the one place where I know most of the people and have someone to talk to—a bit of exercise for my mind."

He used to "coordinate difficulties no matter what it was" for several restaurants. For example, if one restaurant had trouble with water power he'd go to the main office, where people remembered him. "So I go over to Bob, one of the older guys, who is now a foreman. I used to meet him at the Trade and Labour Council. 'How are ya doing there?' I'd say. 'What is it, Avram?' he'd ask. 'Well I'm supposed to ask you this and that and the other thing. And I'm not going to ask you, the hell with it.' So he'd say, 'Well you're the brain, OK? Whenever you want anything you just give a shout. No worry about anything, everything will be fixed,' because he recalled the time I had to put him in his place, you know."

"You *used* to do that. What happened?"

Avram replies: "Well, George (the boss) retired, new management took over and things changed entirely." Avram explains that his skills weren't well understood, weren't really needed in the same way, because a lot of the help now were students or non-union, and management can get away with anything. He still has a job if he wants it, but the relationships are so different that he wants "to get the hell out of there and find something to do on a regular basis."

He is looking. In the meantime he does some volunteer work, most recently at a public school near his home, helping to teach children effective reading. It helps him practise his French, and the teachers value his wartime experience with language classes for refugees. The rest of the week he goes down to the Exhibition grounds and hangs around the snack bar with old friends, although "the history we share is dying off," and many have health problems and can't get down as often. There are more young people now, and they don't know him, or his story, and most of them "aren't really that interested anyway." He still watches every football game at the stadium; they're "just my cup of tea. I get in because I know the people on the gate."

Sometimes he goes to Montreal for a break and loves it when he recognizes someone walking along St. Catherine Street.

"He'll be coming the other way, and I'm saying to myself, 'Oh boy, what's his name, what's his name?' and then I say, 'Hey, where the hell've you been!' And then I'll remember."

"He's an old union member?"

"No, no—I've played football with him. An old worker I'd remember right away."

"What's the difference?"

"I would have a way of knowing how, when, or where. They speak to you differently."

"In French?"

"No, because the relationship is different. We did a lot together, the same situations, the same problems, remember the same things. We have a lot to talk about."

Being in familiar situations with people whose work experience he can share is becoming more rare and so doesn't really help with what he says is really throwing him off— forgetting appointments even when he marks them down. He says his sister is "not so good," and he worries that loss of memory is in the family and that he might be developing Alzheimer's. He remembers his appointments down at the "Ex" but otherwise there's nothing to remember because "Where I am now, I don't *do* anything."

Even marking things down reminds him that he's forgetting things. Like Callum, he hasn't got a "simple system" for remembering home-based activities. And his wife never fails to notice his lapses. When she sees that he forgets something "it throws her," as Avram says, and she keeps harping on it. "She'll say things like, 'How did you forget dear, I just mentioned it half an hour ago.' It's easy for her; she was brought up to it. She knows where everything is—she put them there! It's like she's rubbing it in. Then I think that I don't know how right I am and I lose confidence and get downhearted."

It's clear that Avram has few people to talk with about his life, then or now, and I ask him if he's ever written down any of his experiences in the labour movement, like a memoir. He hasn't, and he is very doubtful that he could, because it would mean "going way back in history, and that would be a lot of work and a difficult job." He would need help with the research and that's not his world. "That's the trouble," he says, "who would help you, who would be interested to do that?"

Back in Harness

His tone of helplessness, even hopelessness, strikes me, so I push a bit. I suggest that someone doing research in political science at the university might love to sit and talk with him, just listen as he reminisces, as I've been doing. I said that they'd know a lot more than I did and offer to ask around among my colleagues.

He replies that he doesn't think he would be "successful in that endeavour you know, in relating, in putting it all together." I assure him that whoever was working with him would help him with that. "Because they'd be interested in your stories, full of the images and actions of those times. You remember so much, and you're so sharp about how things happened, how things were related and the whole process … Stories like yours can disappear unless someone records them, which is a shame, because then they're lost to history."

Avram turns down my suggestion, kindly, but firmly (he is, after all, an experienced negotiator)—it isn't "his cup of tea," not the way he "trained his mind." We talk about the many skills he has developed as a union organizer and negotiator. I suggest that there are still places where he can put those skills to use, and he looks at me quizzically. I ask him if he's ever talked with the director of the seniors' centre where we'd had the memory workshop, about organizing and leading some of the groups they hold. He is quite surprised and says he doesn't think of himself as "being on that level," with an incomplete high school education.

"Hey, Avram!" I reply. "You're a problem solver, you've got all those people skills, you're diplomatic [as I've just experienced], you've led plenty of groups, you speak three languages, and you're used to all the emotions—people getting angry or upset—that can crop up, you can handle all that. I think you'd do a great job."

"It's an idea, I'll think about it. I'd like to tackle something."

I tell him about the life review classes at Ryerson College (now University), where groups of six or so people look back over their lives, have a look at what's been important, or not, and that he might enjoy such a group, could easily lead one.

"And," I add, "the centre is thinking of starting one, but they need a leader."

"It's possible," he replies.

I go on to describe the group a good friend of mine is leading and the fun they are having. "She just makes sure people keep on track, and everyone has time to tell their stories. *That* sounds like just your cup of tea."

"That sounds more like it, all right."

Avram joined a life review group at Ryerson and went on to lead several groups at the seniors' centre. The director was delighted. Now Avram is negotiating relationships and solving problems, "understanding the backgrounds of all sides, not just the immediate problem"—busy "maintaining this, that, and the other."

A Note from Avram

Leading these groups has got me into a little reading, which I never had time for before. You probably know about this guy Doidge[2] but I didn't and he sure has hit the nail on the head for me. He's got these seven key points that once you remember them can be a big help with how you understand what's going on in your life.

Memory is critical to learning. Well that seems obvious. It's just that once I was stuck at home what was there to learn?

Motivation and challenge alter the brain. What's so challenging about being around home? I wasn't so much in the mood to do anything there and had to get out. Once I got out I was OK.

Plasticity can be positive or negative. So, like I said you get stuck in a rut, like those coconuts at work who wouldn't take on anything new. It's like they had rusted brains.

Brains can change at all stages of life, so they are vulnerable to physical and emotional shock. I was sure stressed out with those stubborn guys arguing on all sides, and then with thinking I was losing it when I had to stop work.

Changes happen gradually. I guess it took me awhile to move into another level, but it doesn't

---

[2] Dr. Norman Doidge, *The Brain That Changes Itself* (London: Penguin, 2007). See also Posit Science http://www.positscience.com/ and Brain Fitness Gym http://www.thebrainfitnessgym.com/ websites.

seem so different what I'm doing now than when I was working with the unions ... everyone has their problems no matter what their stage in life.

Exercise assists brain change and learning. There's a class at the centre. It's not football, but I wouldn't be too good at that now anyway. We go out afterwards for a coffee and to chew the fat; it's almost like old times, like I used to do at the Ex., only with new heads.

Initially, changes in the brain are temporary; repetition is essential. I guess you get used to doing it and it's like you always have. There's a lot of stuff I don't need anymore, but that doesn't bother me now.

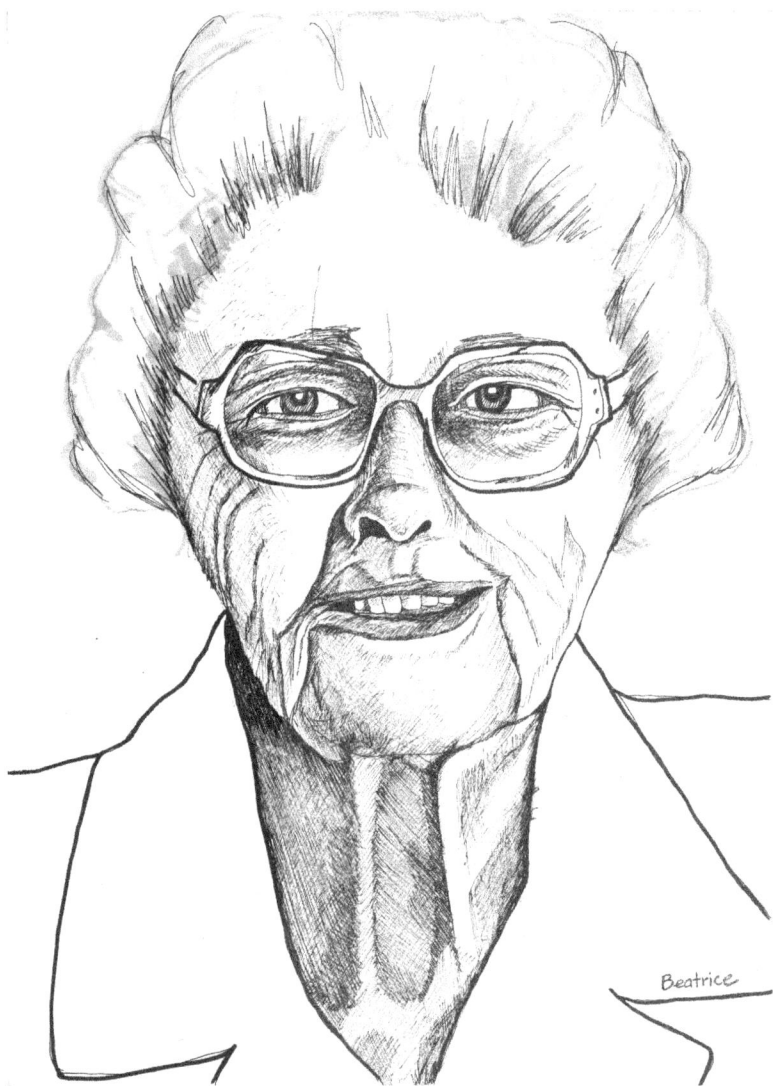

Beatrice

The Faces of Our Dreams Are Still Around Us: Beatrice's Story

"I have to be bolder than I ever was."

Beatrice's scarred little face and her lovely full mouth twisted to one side is a shock at first and I am glad she had forewarned me. But her brown eyes still dance a welcome under curling white hair as we hug each other. I had heard from her daughter Isobel that she'd had a serious automobile accident and written to ask if she would like a visitor but didn't hear back for a year. Eventually she replied, telling me that she had moved to a seniors' residence and would love to see me, suggesting that we meet there. She refused to have lunch out as a "waste of money"—she'd lost her sense of taste, and besides, she "had limited mobility."

"You're so like your mother," she exclaims. "The minute I look at you I remember her, how we would not see each other for years and have the same relationship when we met." She shows me around "The Manor," and my heart aches for the people, mostly women, sitting alone in the lounge staring into space, some murmuring to themselves. And it aches for her. She must have sensed my distress, because when we reach her room she looks at me and says, "You're wondering why I'm here, aren't you?"

"It doesn't look much like your kind of place."

"Well, I've got a roommate again," she smiles (she was my mother's roommate at university). "But I made sure she'd be out when you came so that we'd have time to ourselves."

"Are you OK with this?"

"Partly Living": The Manor

"Well, I wasn't at first. But there was no choice. There are no single rooms, and that's really a good thing, otherwise people would be alone at night. The nurses come in, but you don't hear them. You see, after the accident I was crying all the time because I couldn't look after myself. When I lost my sense of taste I stopped eating, it didn't seem worthwhile. And if something spilled on the floor I couldn't get down to clean it. Isobel came on weekends, but then she moved to Toronto with her children for a better job. I had a TV and radio with a tape recorder, a stereo, and lots of books, and I'd just sit there and cry. A social worker came to visit and said it was a depression, and I said, 'To hell with this, I've got to move.' That's when I decided I wanted to live. I didn't, after the accident; I wondered why I hadn't died."

She chose a seniors' residence in the town she grew up in, thinking that she'd at least know a few people and there would be some company, something to give her the will to live. Now that she has things more in perspective, she realizes that the move was probably a mistake, because "they're no different than when I grew up, just as stodgy as they ever were. People know everything you do. That might seem friendly, but really they're not, if you don't fit the mould."

The nursing home provides the necessities. Meals are at set times, so the staff know you are there, and she has to eat. At first, she thought that she'd go crazy: "There's no one here who is interested in the things I am, hardly anyone even talks."

Beatrice and my mother talked a lot. They attended University College at the University of Toronto in the early 1920s, and after a somewhat rocky start they became fast friends. Beatrice hadn't known that if you wanted a single room you had to ask for it, and the dean at Queen's Hall residence, seeing that she came from a small town and "needed the experience," had put her in a double room.

"We went along the hall, and eventually we got down to my room. Grace [my mother] was there, and she said, 'This is my bed, and this is my dresser, and this is my cupboard, and the rest is yours.' So I said, 'Fine,' and she didn't say anything else. She went away by herself, and I said to myself, 'Well, OK, you can't help it. Here we are, and if she doesn't like me I can't help it, and she can't help it.' So we were on that footing for quite a while. Eventually we got so we could talk to each other in the room, and we had the same ideas about everything, and one day by accident we went shopping together and got back, and Grace said, 'You're the only person I ever liked shopping with.' And I said, 'Well, I liked shopping with you too.' We got along well together after that. She talked about one boyfriend she had where she grew up that had hurt her badly. I happened to know him and that he had hurt a girl in my high school badly too—he always pretended you were his girl until he found another. She'd never really talked to anyone about it; after that we talked about other things that had happened."

Both Beatrice and my mother grew up in small towns and felt that they had escaped to a much more interesting world when they left for university. There was so much to see and do: tea at Mary Jane's Tea Room, a "full-meal" baked apple at Murray's Restaurant when they were broke, more bookstores than they'd ever dreamed of, the Jewish and Chinese districts, poetry readings in candlelit rooms, political meetings and interesting men, the endlessly fascinating stacks of the library. And although neither of them drank or smoked, they enjoyed the pleasurable rebellion of not going to church. "I didn't really know why Grace was against it until years later, when we confessed to each other that her parents and my grandparents were Plymouth Brethren, which was socially unacceptable. She used to say that the PBs made the Presbyterians seem like Rabelaisians. I miss her a lot and wonder what we'd be talking about now."

I ask why it had been so long before she'd told me she'd moved, and she says that she just couldn't talk to anyone, even Isobel.

"I'm sorry I didn't smarten up and realize there must have been something wrong."

"I probably wouldn't have gotten back to you any sooner. I felt pretty awful. And then I began to see, looking at the company around me, that physical problems are not as bad as mental breakdown, although mine was more an emotional thing than mental—as if they could be separated. With physical breakdown, you're just sitting and staring, you've lost any connection to life." She thinks her level of activity and interests are pretty good, considering her disability. She has adjusted to having to do other things, and tries not to resent it—after all, "a lot of people can't even read anymore." She tells me that they are taking a survey to find out what the residents can do. I ask why they don't ask the residents themselves, and she replies with a shrug that "they don't know."

"But *you* know."

"Well, I can still get on the bus, the one with the special stairs, and go uptown, go to the library, shop anytime I'm up to it. I'm talking about my roommate who is 91. Even with her hearing aid she can only hear her radio when it's on so loud that I can't stay in the room. Doesn't ever use earphones. She is a nice person, I feel sorry, but there's nothing I can do. If I'm not there she just sits, like the people in the lobby, in the same way they just sit and smoke a lot and stare ahead. It's depressing, to say the least. You try to talk to them and cheer them up, but what they need is a family, and you see they don't have family."

"And you have Isobel and the children. Can they get here often now that they've moved?"

"Isobel manages once a month, and the children when they can. The older ones are working now, and it's hard for them to remember that they can't just run over the way they used to. They have their own interests. I don't complain, they just need reminders now and again."

Beatrice is very clear about what it's like to feel old. At 81, her body is old, but not her mind. She can't see, hear, taste, or walk as well. Can't do anything the way she used to. Can't even sew. "This isn't just me, because there are all the people of the residence to go by. [She's still a researcher at heart!] Even things you did well take a lot longer. You feel frustrated. If you want to walk down to the lake it would normally be a five-minute walk; now I have to allow half an hour to get down there and half an hour to get back. You have to plan whatever you're doing. Normally you would walk downtown and do three things and zip back and do the washing and the ironing, but now you have to take the whole day to do those three things and not get mad at the whole thing."

"Time has slowed down to keep you company."

"It seems that way. Depressing. You can't do what you used to be able to do. Doesn't seem any reason for it. Just slowing down, wearing out, you realize it won't come back." She thinks that the accident accelerated the natural physical slowing down of aging, but she doesn't feel different or older mentally.

"Is being old what you expected?"

"No, I didn't think you'd continue to think young."

"That's a surprise for you?"

"Yes, a surprise."

"Because you'd picked up the idea along the way that older people didn't think very well?"

"No, that's not true. Just that you have to keep reminding yourself that your body's old. It doesn't do what you want it to do!"

I ask her what thinking young means to her, and she replies that it's "just part of her," thinks for a minute, and then gives me an example of reading in the local paper that a new "Y" (YWCA) would be built and thinking how nice it would be to use it, with all the new advantages, especially the pool. She'd always loved swimming. "Then I began to see—what could I use? Unless they had special ways for disabled people to help them get in the pool. This is what I mean."

"Because your old enthusiasms are still there?"

"Still there, yes. You don't turn off, you adapt. You say to yourself that maybe you can't do everything, but you can do something, like finding out if there's a way for disabled people to get into the pool."

"Then you have to get logical and reasonable," I say. "You make a face when I say that, you don't like it" *laughing together* "—who would? But you do that, don't you? You continue to do the things you've always liked, like walking and swimming, only more slowly. Like the 83-year-old woman in May Sarton's book *At Seventy* who had perfected the art of gardening at a slow tempo so that it was like a meditation."

She remembers visiting the wonderful garden near Southampton on the Bruce Peninsula with Isobel and the man tending it who still made beautiful carvings at 90. I ask her if she thinks of herself in the same way, with the full days she has. She says she will hear people say, "So and so is wonderful for her age" or is "wonderful for what she does," and thinks to herself that she's not so bad. But other people don't tell *her* that.

"Maybe because you have simply continued to do what you have always done and don't make a fuss about it."

"I think that is what it is, alright!"

"So people expect you to be wonderful!"

She tells me how her grandfather, who lived with them, was the only old person she knew very well while she was growing up. She was too young to wonder how he felt when he started to slow down, or what he thought about growing old, or if he still thought of himself as young, the way she does now. It never occurred to her, because whatever her parents were doing they just kept on doing until they died. Her mother kept on going to meetings at the church and her book club, her father played bridge and poker and gardened until he began to suffer from a mild dementia two years before he died. "He couldn't play cards anymore, but he spent hours tending the garden and seemed happy right to the end."

"Your models of what old people are like were people who slowed down but didn't give up. You don't, do you?"

"No, I don't. After the accident I was unconscious for a week, and when I came to I wanted them to just let me go. I thought 'Why do doctors have to keep you going?' Then my brother died well before I was able to walk again, and he was eight years younger than I was, and I wondered if I was supposed to die too. And I didn't. Why didn't I? You don't know that your life is planned out for you, but I do think that you do things sometimes for a reason. You wouldn't have planned it that way, but you go ahead and do it."

"Are you glad you didn't die?"

"I was thinking about that one day, and I began to think of all the interesting things I've done since then, like Elderhostel. So I'm glad I didn't. But it was close."

I mention that although I hadn't been injured nearly as badly as she had, I had fractured the vertebrae in my back a few years earlier, had to do a lot of adapting myself, and was usually pretty uncomfortable, adding that I'd had my days when I wondered whether it was worthwhile to keep on going.

"Are you comfortable sitting there?" Beatrice asks.

"I'm fine. I just wiggle a lot to change my position. And you know, since I started writing again, I've realized, the way you have, that I have had a head start on what you have to do to adjust to aging."

"So, it's not all bad. On your good days, that is!" she says.

"That's right, but then you know all about that."

Seeing how relatively well she is in comparison to her neighbours makes her realize that it's not age or disability that has you "going downhill," it's that the people around you don't share any of your interests. So it's "hard to find anything to do in the present, anything that's worth remembering; that's why old people talk about the past a lot, that's often all they have. I'm really fortunate that I can still get on the bus, although it's hard to make up my mind to do it. The others here, they're trapped. They couldn't do anything for themselves even if they wanted to. And most of them don't know any better, don't know what they want. Why would they? Where would they have learned it?"

After she moved to the nursing home, Beatrice thought it "was a pretty stupid move for the first few weeks. I had to get torn out of London first, and the way of life there, into the way of life at the residence, where there isn't one single person in the 142 residents who is interested in learning."

"It must have been dreadfully lonely."

Reaching Out

"It was. It was crazy-making. I got to wondering if I wasn't the one out of line, until I remembered I'd always been different from my classmates when I was growing up." Then she joined Elderhostel and picked up where she'd left off at the university. While those early student days were not a resource for personal or social change at the time, they had been a brief "coming out" for her, because she "didn't have to hide as much as you do in a small town." However, during her married life she had to "put her intellectual life on hold again because my husband did not approve, and there was no time anyway." She had been interested in theology and anthropology all her life but never had the opportunity to study them, didn't even know that she wanted to until she took a course in theology at Elderhostel and thought, "Oh, wow, this is it."

The next year she took a correspondence course in theology from the University of Waterloo. Archaeology was part of that, and then astronomy. It was wonderful to know that she was just as bright as she ever was. She took courses and passed exams, even when she had to take time out to have a pacemaker put in. "There is nothing the matter with my memory," she states firmly. The classes are important not only for the excitement of new information, but also for the intellectual stimulation of meeting people who have similar interests and are eager to talk about them. Like everyone else whom I talked with, she knows that "you need other people, because talking and sharing are crucial to memory and mental health." (Alice talks about "bogging down," Lev about "deteriorating," Rebecca about losing the zest for life, Miriam and Meyer about becoming too "in-grown" or getting out of touch and becoming "selfish," as Emma would say.)

Beatrice calls it "going downhill," and, like so many women then and now, she did wonder for a while if she was being selfish to spend so much time on herself, going to classes and seminars. However, when her disability worsened and she could no longer go to Elderhostel, she had proved to herself that her mind "was still as good as ever," despite her physical condition, and decided to learn to use the computer so she could write the weekly newsletter for The Manor. Remembering daily household chores and appointments was no longer a concern, because "all that is looked after here." The "everyday task" in a nursing home is the struggle to stay active, alert, and involved, so that "you can talk about something else besides the weather." As a way of remembering her life and feeling alive, she not only keeps in touch with her family ("for the history") but also takes on other interests. She had been active in the Girl Guide movement for years and reconnected as one of its senior advisers through a good friend who was a guide captain when she was guide captain leader. She lives a block away from Beatrice, who usually stays there for supper— a welcome reprieve from the blandness of institutional meals. Beatrice serves tea and coffee after the exercise program, volunteers at the library on Books on Wheels days—the chief librarian, who comes in three days a week, is also a friend. The administrator, whom she knew as a little boy, asked her to become a part of a new Resident's Council, and "that takes up an hour."

"That's one advantage of coming back to your hometown, I guess."

"Oh, I guess so. And then you see, when I began to do things around the place I felt better. And the nurses are wonderful. You can talk to any of them, unless they're terribly busy. They're very understanding and seem to talk to you as a friend. I know they're trained to do that, but it's nice to be able to stop in to the office or the craft room for a chat. But the residents?! There's one person I used to know, she married one of the boys in the group I used to dance and skate with—I don't think they have things like that now, where if you went alone a couple would see you home. Her husband died three years ago, and she went into shock. Apparently is still in shock, living entirely in the past. I thought she'd like to go to Elderhostel. But no."

If she didn't take the initiative to make connections in town, as well as in the residence, she "would just have to live the life of the residence, which is not a life at all." Knowing how connected physical well-being is to learning and memory, she objected to the quality of life in the home and decided to do more research into the alternative and complementary health care that helped her so much, so that she "will not be the only one to benefit." She knows from her own experience that "the doctors are not interested in the chronically ill or disabled even when you're not old. They just want to give you a pill and forget about it. I mean they want to forget about you, and you're supposed to forget about yourself too. But how do you forget you're in pain? I don't want to spend my life in a drug haze." She is the "house member of a patient's advocate's group and bugs the board" about environmentally healthy measures such as not using strong chemicals to clean and serving more nutritious food.

Taking this kind of leadership role is not natural for Beatrice, because she was never "trained to do that at home or at school, even at the university. If there was an active Seniors' Society in town, I guess they'd need a leader. If they want me I'll be it, but I'd rather just be a member."

"It seems to me that you have it all there, but you hold yourself back."

"Yep."

"And that's not new for you, is it?"

"No."

"Maggie Kuhn says that many older people, especially women, are unused to thinking that they have anything worthwhile to contribute. You're nodding your head in agreement. Does that mean you think that way about yourself?"

"Yes. Yes I do."

"And that they are not used to being asked their opinions."

"Well, you know that you have an opinion, but you don't think it matters to anyone else, and so mostly you keep it to yourself. Except that now I've been speaking out a little." She describes the members of the Women's Auxiliary, who do things for residents thinking they know what they want. She had publicly disagreed with them in meetings, "which didn't go down too well." To be so outspoken was also new for her, and she wishes now she'd taken a course in public speaking. She has looked around locally, hasn't found one, and is amused at people's reactions to an old woman's asking about it.

"Giving yourself a pat on the back for doing as well as you have after the accident doesn't come easily, does it? It's hard for you to think about yourself in those terms."

She agrees, saying that some people think she has an inferiority complex but she thinks not. She's just herself, neither inferior nor superior. She and Grace never thought of bolstering each other up. Grace was a bit undermining of herself. They criticized other people instead—as a way of making themselves feel better, she guessed. She learned how to keep her opinions to herself in school. If you wanted to go out with a man or be invited anywhere, that's what you did. Most of the professors didn't ask you anyway. After she married, her husband was very critical of her, putting her down all the time. She didn't know "why he needed to do that"; she'd worked very hard and felt she was a good wife and mother. And so, when the children were older, she left her husband. He was very angry, "That was a disgrace, you see. For him." That is all she ever said about her marriage, other than making a face whenever I happen to mention her husband. She tells me that leaving him forced her out of her shell. "I never thought I was any good. Had never had a good job, never made any major decisions like that, except to be married, and that wasn't a decision, girls got married. That's what they did. After the divorce I had to make my own decisions, and it was good for me. Painful though."

"And now you have to be more assertive to survive in the nursing home."

"Yes, I certainly do."

I tell her that reminded me of a book by Barbara Myerhoff, *Number Our Days*, about a group of elderly Jewish nursing-home residents in California. They had emigrated from Europe to the United States—California, I think—to give their children a better life, but those same children grew up embarrassed about their parents' European accents and foreign ways. The author found that it was the old people who were vociferous in their complaints who did not deteriorate mentally, and that it seems as if Beatrice has been more assertive, like them.

"How's that?"

"Well, you went to university when not many women did. You left an abusive marriage and made a life, bringing up adolescent children on your own. Whether consciously or unconsciously, you decided to live after the accident. You kept on learning and went to Elderhostel when you knew you had to do something to survive in the seniors' residence. And now that you can't do that anymore, you've found—even invented—other things to do that are interesting, and make a contribution as well."

"Well! Well, you have to have someone to care for, to make a contribution. And you need something to look forward to."

I ask what bolsters her up, saying that I didn't hear her criticizing other people now to make herself feel better. Laughing, she responds that she doesn't have to do that anymore. She thinks about nice things that have happened, nice places she's been to. People she's known, like my mother, and their friends—"that whole gang, they were an interesting group of women, and lots of fun too. I don't think about things like my marriage, or the accident, although that's harder because my body reminds me all the time, especially when I'm tired or not busy."

"Sort of creeps up on you unawares."

"Yes, it does."

The Joys of Remembering
Staying Alive

For Beatrice, reminiscence was not a life review, in Martha's sense of making something meaningful of her life, or looking for meaning in an overall picture, like Meyer. For her, remembering the past was a way of feeling alive, of remembering that she has had a full life and of connecting that life to who she is now. "People criticize old people for remembering the past more than the present, but I don't know about that. I think it's very nice to remember people you used to like and things you used to do. I get a great deal of enjoyment, especially when I'm lying in bed and can't sleep."

"What else would you do with your experiences if you can't think about them?"

"That's just it, nobody else can do them, or they'd just be lies."

"Like somebody else writing your autobiography? That has me wondering what you think about what I'm doing. How will we know that it's you?"

"That's different, you're doing research, and then you're writing up a story, but you're not doing my remembering. Sometimes Isobel does that."

"Children thinking they know more about you than you do!"

"Right! But I ignore it; I know she wants to be helpful."

"You mentioned thinking about the past as a way to help you sleep. How do you do that?"

"Well, I focus on a topic for the night. You just think about what you're going to remember. I've done a lot of different things, lived a lot of different lives, so to speak."

"Some people focus on sounds or sights or smells. What's your particular way?"

She likes to think about the places she's been, her university days, the sports she's played. After a while she'll think, "I used to know that boy quite well, what is it we used to do?" Once she starts, spontaneous memory takes over. Pictures and scenes keep on unrolling, the layers peel away, and things she hasn't planned on will pop up, and she'll start to think about that, how she went dancing, "and if he had a car or not. And you remember what he looked like and what you talked about, and then you wonder why you never saw him anymore, and that usually comes back too. And, well, different things that trigger your memory. Coming back to my home town has triggered a lot. I have a pictorial image of it. And then, after a while, I'll go to sleep and I'll dream. I dream in colour."

She tries to forget the bad dreams, dreams of when somebody said something nasty, or hurt her feelings, thinking to herself, "Oh, well, it's only a dream." And she's had some wonderful dreams, usually about singing, dancing, and swimming. She's very certain that her reminiscence is social and sensory—"organized," as she says—according to various places and people and interactions that she visualizes. As she tells me about it, she laughs and says, "Sometimes I have a struggle to stay connected among so many lives, so it's good to talk about it sometimes, because no one knows them now but me."

"There is nobody left who is a part of those memories."

"That's right. See, when I talk to you, you knew some of those people, even if you were only a child and then a teenager, and that makes it seem more real and not just a dream. And, of course, your mother. I remember the time she talked about joining a sorority. We got invitations, and she had quite a few, and she had quite a time deciding what to do. She talked it over with that teacher who helped her go to university."

"Elizabeth Kingston. We got together for tea every year after mother died, until she died a few years ago when she was 92."

"Oh, did she? I couldn't join one, because my father couldn't afford it. Or that's what he said. But Grace did, and I think it helped her a lot."

"I didn't know she'd joined a sorority. Elizabeth must have helped her with that too, because mother's father didn't want her to go to university and didn't contribute a cent. That story has triggered *my* memory! What else triggers yours?"

"Oh, familiar sights and sounds. Buying something and putting it where it's supposed to be. I like to know where everything is, what's on each individual shelf. There's a short-term memory and a long-term memory, and the short-term memory can put things into the long term. The things you want to remember you tell your short-term memory to remember it, to put it in long-term memory. That works for me."

"That's so wonderfully practical!" I laughed. You trust your memory the way Emma does. And you pay attention." She replies that she writes things down as well, but that she never has remembered names, a habit that has nothing to do with old age.

"I remember the minister we had, one time after a meeting I chaired we were shaking hands with everyone, and he said how wonderful it was I remembered names. But, you see, I wasn't remembering their names, I was remembering their faces, and as they went out I would smile and say good night, and he thought I was remembering their names. I realized the best thing to do when you forget is to ask about how they're doing. If it was one of the Girl Guides, I would remember *them*, but not their name. Otherwise you just say nothing." Beatrice thought that remembering and forgetting "is a bit like housecleaning; you can't keep everything, you're bound to throw out some of the things you're going to want."

"And keep some of the things you don't?"

"That's right, the bad memories. I always think I have a bad memory when I can't get rid of that stuff."

Sensory Memory

If she's not deliberately trying to remember something specific, it's usually something sensory that evokes memory for her, like seeing a piece of furniture and thinking, "'I know that plaid from way back,' and then I'll think, 'Where did I know it?' And remember that. That sort of thing. Or it might be something somebody says, or seeing someone dancing on TV. And I always watch the skating, and remember my skating days."

"So colour evokes a particular memory. It's the senses again, isn't it? For you, colour, and actions like swimming and dancing."

"I can't just sit there and not have a thought. I don't know how people do that."

This was an interesting juxtaposition. I say senses and actions, and she picks up on action as a part of thinking. I ask her how she "thinks" colour or activities, and she tells me that these kinds of memories and dreams would be better expressed in painting and drawing. She is keeping a journal, writing to that "other person" she talks with when there's no one else around, but she tells me that she'd "be ashamed to read what I wrote and would tear it up."

"Because it's too intimate, too 'in your face,' as the kids would say?"

"I'm sorry I never learned to draw, because what I do like to do is watercolour, and rarely do. Because, you see, I can't draw." I tell her about the ways I've learned to work in pastels and watercolour that don't depend on making something representational, that I'd found that making a recognizable object doesn't matter too much. And she replied, "It does to me. I try, but I can't express how I feel in a drawing."

"I know what you mean, I was really scared the first time I was asked to draw something in a class, because of my sister being an artist, and my thinking I couldn't be. When the instructor asked us to use our non-dominant hand as a way to get rid of what we thought we should be doing, that helped free me up." Beatrice agreed that we're all brought up in a left-brain culture.

I went on to say that I'd read *Drawing on the Right Side of the Brain* and that it had liberated me some more. She doubts if the book will be in the local library, and I remind her of interlibrary loan and offer to send her a copy if she can't get it that way. "It pulled a part of my brain I wasn't used to using as much. But, you know, it's just like what you do when you're reminiscing and dreaming, remembering the past in all its vividness and vitality and then making connections to your life now. That's a different way of remembering than what you need for learning facts, acquiring information, and so forth. What do you think memory is for?"

"That's a startling question. I don't think you could live without memory. It's life. What has been and is and is going to be. I don't see how, if a person who doesn't have memory, she could live in any sense except physically. I always have thoughts. If I can't sleep—you have to do something with your mind—I know I'll fall asleep eventually, but instead of counting sheep, I'll count what I did on all the New Year's Eves. I have a perfectly wonderful time seeing all these people. I had no memory whatsoever of getting there and back. So what I tried to do in my mind was think: 'How did I get there?'" She tells me how she remembered she was on the train, and then the conductor's wake-up call, and remembering it was for the wrong station.

"The train, the conductor, and so on, are they in colour?"

"Oh, yes. Always in colour. And I see them moving—like the conductor swaying down the corridor, how the wheels look going around more slowly, and how I would wake up and look out the window. You know, if the young knew how important memory was going to be they'd take care to make good ones!"

"Like you have! Remembering in pictures, activities, through relationships. It's very sensory—pictorial and kinaesthetic, isn't it? Like you're reconstructing sensory and social impressions that way, and then you decide what you will remember and forget."

"It is really. I trust my mind."

She loves remembering in vivid sensory and kinaesthetic detail yet values her mental capacities even more. As was the case with Miriam and Lev, Beatrice's body had let her down so badly, and was so painful, that she really didn't want to focus on the physical, even to acknowledge how important the sensory was to her memory, as Meyer and Miriam could do. But for all of them, mental breakdown was much worse than physical breakdown. Fully aware of her social and educational privileges, Beatrice doesn't feel socially or physically privileged now. She is in physical and social pain all the time. But she is thankful for her education, because she sees all around her the difference an education can make to living a decent old age. She is grateful that the accident did not damage her mind, that she "can still use and take pleasure in it," as she always had.

"Like my friend Meyer said, 'You've trained your mind.'"

"I didn't really know I had until after the accident. I think I'm past getting Alzheimer's. I've looked into it on the computer, and I'm probably too old now. It's going to be something else."

Citizen of the Year

Beatrice found an Elderhostel at Cambrian College in Sudbury that "catered more to disabled people," saw Science North from a wheelchair while she was there, and "had a wonderful time." She became president of the Resident's Council and belonged to the Regional Executive, both of which met monthly. And I laughed as I imagined her "speaking out" pleasantly, quietly, and very firmly. She went to the Provincial Annual Meeting of Homes for the Aged at the Convention Centre in Hamilton and visited homes in Barrie, Durham, Owen Sound, and Shelbourne and wrote a report on what she found, calling it *The Observations of an Insider.* "I would like to have said 'inmate' but didn't think that would be useful," she commented to me. And I saw her crooked little smile and those raised eyebrows expressing what she didn't say.

"Isobel is working in Hamilton and can get up more often, the children can drive up now that they're older, and that's such a pleasure. I see them almost as much as when we lived together when they were little. I still swim twice a week [Did she talk them into putting in handicap access? I forgot to ask.], and have rides on my tricycle that the family gave me for my last birthday. I visit friends and go to the odd meeting. It is as much fun as possible, I expect."

But she doesn't mention the honour she received as her home town's Citizen of the Year, awarded for her many years of service to the community. (Neither she nor my mother would ever have drawn attention to any of their achievements.) I saw the write-up in a Toronto paper under a smiling photograph of her dressed in a rose-coloured sweater, a pearl necklace and earrings, holding a bouquet of daisies. I wrote to congratulate her, saying that I marvelled how she "had found ways to keep on doing what she had always done." She replied that the honour had been a complete surprise: "At first I thought they'd made a mistake because I don't think I've done any more than anyone else. I've been thinking of Grace a lot these days and your letter reminded me that the last time we saw each other we had planned to go to the next UC reunion and have fun. I still miss her a lot."

Roommates

The Dean said small-town girls need
company. So, G and I stood at the door
and she said, "This is my bed, this is my dresser,
and this is my cupboard. The rest is yours."
"Fine," I said. Then she went away.
"Well, OK," I said to the air, "if she doesn't like
me
I can't help it. And she can't help it."
Eventually we got talking in the room—
we had the same ideas
about everything. One day by accident we
went shopping together.
"You're the only person I ever liked shopping
with,"
she said. "Well, I like shopping with you too."
We got along well after that. Talked
about everything. Wakeful in bed
I remember the boyfriend that hurt her badly
she'd never told anyone about, the dances we'd
never
been allowed, picnics where the highway
hums now … Two old women talking before
sleep.

Epilogue: A World of Wonders

We all become stories. Do we create ourselves through telling our stories?

Do the stories we tell reveal how the stories we are born into create us?

Beliefs and Values

All living beings proceed through a series of life stages that appear to be biologically inevitable and that share many predictable characteristics. But, as Miriam said, "We are made up of the times we are born into." In every generation, in every culture, human beings grow up with beliefs and values about home, education, work, and what follows that mould what they accept as true and shape how they live. Intellect, emotions, and spirit, all borne by our physical body, receive values and beliefs within these places and the notion that they are separate spheres may obscure the reality of their intricate individual and social relationships.

As we age, we live uneasily within and across these categories. Then gradually, or suddenly, we become "old," as our society defines it, in beliefs that inform regulations and programs about pensions, life insurance, retirement, post-retirement occupations, seniors' programs, elder support, long-term care, and the like, where the unique potential of older age can fall victim to the common assumption that as elders "fall apart" (in Lev's words), they become useless, irrelevant, and helpless.

In western culture we are usually dependent on our physical condition and mental faculties for a sense of self-worth, independence, and connection to community. Since aging bodies do slow down and exhibit signs of wear and tear, older people can feel discouraged and dispirited when they are perceived to be at "the end of the line" and can readily be led to believe that there are no further vistas to explore and nothing further to contribute.

What I have learned throughout my long life and from the many people I have talked to, some of whom have told their stories in this book, is how often in our lives we cross the boundaries that mark what happens and who does what in home, education, work, retirement, and old age. Sometimes planfully, sometimes inadvertently, often with more or less resistance from our various social contexts, including our families. *We All Become Stories* shows us many of the different ways elders deal with the inevitable consequences of physical aging, yet challenge the "predictable"—conventional notions of aging and where the old belong and what they should do—creating testaments to the exceptional opportunities inherent in this stage of life. Clearly, traditional assumptions about the behaviour and feelings appropriate to particular places and stages of life may be socially convenient, but they may not be individually relevant. Why does this wisdom not pass from one generation to the next, when it could be so useful in dealing with similar struggles?

Challenging Boundaries

This book is not a political, social, or psychological analysis about what Emma called "the conditions we grow up in." It is a venue for 12 courageous women and men to talk about the ways, places, and occasions in which their social conditions have shaped them and they way they wrestled with, often savoured, life's stages. Their stories are "memory work," narratives of when, where, and how they were able, or not, to transgress the barriers that defined these conditions and their images of themselves and the impact their subversion has on their old age. Theirs are tales of how we grow into our singularity.

Community, Identity and Self-Worth

Whatever ways we have lived within social customs or not, there may come a time when our bodies become more frail and we need more community support. At the same time, vital social networks may diminish or evaporate through the loss of friends and family, and increasing isolation may follow declines in hearing, sight, and mobility. And so opportunities to belong may decrease, and "fitting in" may become more difficult. To sustain a sense of "feeling good about ourselves," many of us choose to pursue more personal interests and learn that solitude can open a place for self-discovery and creativity. As Rivka says, she is better now that she feels herself differently. She has "grown into herself" and become less like her peers and more idiosyncratic, more like "who she is," in order to assure a sense of self.

However, this physical, emotional, and intellectual "closing in" and deepening may take up much of the time and energy we have used to maintain our social relationships. "Paying attention to ourselves," so necessary to our sense of well-being, can create doubt and ambivalence about selves and purposes, as Martha found to her disquiet, as she juggled her own pressing needs with the social connections she considered necessary for her survival. Are we deteriorating, or are we changing to suit a more individualistic, rather than group oriented, identity?

Memory Changes: Differences or Decline?

Callum is certain that our adaptations to changing circumstances are often a matter of what we believe, which comes to us through the language of society's values—if we hear or read something enough we may believe it, and if everyone holds and practises the same maxim, then it must be true. The elders in these stories know and make it clear that they fear intellectual decline far more than physical slowing down or even pain. Their beliefs that memory is cognitive and that memory loss is a sure sign of dementia strikes terror into their hearts because they already associate this stage of life with the inevitable deterioration of all parts of themselves and with their separation from the "real" world of work. In terms of society's norms of independence and usefulness, they can no longer "go it alone," are failing, and will become a social hindrance, as Emma had feared.

Cognitive processes such as accuracy of detail, speed of recall, and linear thinking go hand in hand with youth, career building, and the more "masculine" world of work. These characteristics are also the hallmarks of a rapidly developing and sophisticated technology that can make the aging and their lifelong experiences seem "old" hat: "old" fashioned, obsolete, offering nothing to society. Beatrice knows how important it is to "have something to do, something to contribute and something to look forward to" and learns how to use a computer so she can write the newsletter and stay connected. But Meyer often finds the internet's "so-called wealth" of information shallow and boring, not offering him anything to help him grasp the "big picture"; his knowledge and memory threads now seem slow and lackluster to his more youthful friends.

Accepting Sensory Memory

To our dozen explorers, sensory memory—physical, relational, interdependent— at first either does not seem to be memory or, if it does, appears useless or inefficient— more the domain of the "feminine" world of body and of home. However, through illness, change of status, or new personal goals and passions, some of our elders come to understand that humans are all relational and interdependent: that "the nuts and bolts of everyday life"—the sensory world of relationships, nature, and the messy body—is foundational to existence and to ways of remembering. Miriam said, "I've lived long enough to know what I know: the sensory is the basis of how I remember and of memories—welcome and unwelcome. The language of the old faces reality ... sees how people are unwitting victims of their social and cultural conditions." No one ever really leaves home.

And so we may begin to see that what we need and want to remember and forget changes frequently, whether by force of circumstance, as in Avram's case, or through choice, as in Rebecca's, and are efficient adaptations to evolving physical, social, and intellectual needs. Our memory may not "crumble" as we age; rather what we remember and forget may adjust to serve new physical demands and long-germinating dreams. Adapting to less-than-efficient bodies and changing experiences of memory may be idiosyncratic, distinctive, and interesting. While this reframing can help us to carve out a more satisfying life, it may be difficult to "believe," because it runs "against the grain" and risks condescension and alienation from our communities. We may see it as failure, as Russell did, rather than as accommodation and creativity.

This undermining of essential elements of our daily lives highlights the conundrum of believing that memory is entirely cognitive, yet experiencing its grounding in the sensory and its continuous, lifelong partnering with the cognitive. As with the other paradoxes of aging and memory, disagreeing with prevailing beliefs may mean social alienation—when we can't maintain a sense of integrity and still go along with the crowd.

See and Enjoy

My conversations with the elders in this volume introduced me to the fierce resolve and creativity of the aging and old, whose strength, resilience, determination, faith, and trust in themselves, while they were weathering the slings and arrows that seem to aim particularly at old age, stand me in good stead now that I too am old.

From the vantage point of long-life perspectives such as Alice's, they see that every life stage has its perils and joys, some different, some the same. When we think in this both/and kind of way, rather than living an either/or existence, we can see that we can be frail physically *and* strong in mind and spirit. We can learn to balance our well-earned knowledge of how human relationships function at home, and in the bigger picture. We can treasure and nurture our intellect so that we can choose (only) the resources we need from the wealth of new information and technology—and enjoy them!

At first acknowledging, and then experiencing, how our senses absorb information throughout our lives, information that we store and can remember from within our muscles, bones, and cells, offer us a source of wonder and of strength as we see where we come from, what supports us, and the base from which we build. Tuning in to our sensations, feelings, and the mysteries of the natural world—which have always been there—can be restorative, can bring pleasure and satisfaction, depth and richness, consolation and contentment, along with the aches and pains that will inevitably plague us. Learning from their experiences opened for me an awareness of the sensory and of sensory memory I had never experienced, let alone thought of, which has rewarded, and disturbed, my life and writing ever since.

Their stories also show us how accepting, even welcoming, rather than fearing, the inevitability and necessity of change to the very end holds a kind of gleeful challenge, as we allow things to continue to change so that we see what happens as life runs its course.

It is not just our physical brains that are "plastic." Seeing change, difference, and differentness as creative and highly functional opens up our life stories to ourselves so we can welcome our origins in *all* the worlds we live in.

We are sure to waver in the face of the deep challenges of physical and emotional pain and the disbelief, distrust, and dislike that accompany social constraints such as poverty and isolation. But when we can rise to the challenge of Meyer's "tall order"—bounce back, balance all the conflicting needs and demands, and "pull it off"—our lives can fill with old knowledge, new learning, and connections to "the 'brotherhood' of seeing." May I say "kinship," Meyer?

Then we will all be able to tell our untold stories, and pass on the wisdom of the "past and of the now" from one generation to the next so that younger people will cherish and remember their experiences and memories into their old age and incorporate them in the stories that shape us all.

Author Bio

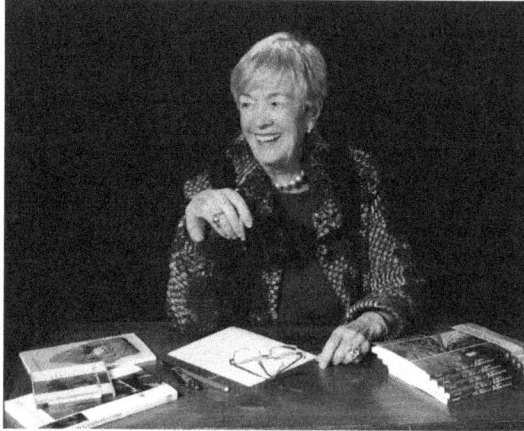

Ann **Elizabeth Carson,** BA and MEd (University of Toronto), Diploma, Arscura School of Art, is a poet, writer, sculptor, and feminist, one of Toronto's Mille Femmes (in the arts) at the 2008 Luminato Festival.

Born in 1929 in Toronto, Ann began writing and publishing in high school and continued during her undergraduate university years and while raising a family. In 1970 she earned a Master's in Adult Education and Counselling at the Ontario Institute for Studies in Education, and she worked for many years as a counsellor, supervisor, and instructor at York University and in a private practice that focused on expressive therapies.

Her published work includes *Shadows Light,* poetry and sculptures (Longboat Alliance, 2005); *My Grandmother's Hair,* about how family stories shape our memories and our lives (Edgar Kent, Dundurn, 2006); *The Risks of Remembrance,* new poems (Words Indeed, 2010); and *We All Become Stories* (Blue Denim Press, 2013). Selections from and reviews of Ann's books and presentations have appeared from Maine to Manitoulin Island and Vancouver.

Ann leads workshops in how the arts create a new perspective in how we see ourselves and our world. She enjoys reading and presenting her work in collaborative events with other writers, artists, dancers, and musicians, as well as with professionals in adult education and health care.

Writing and sculpting full-time in Toronto and on Manitoulin Island, Ann loves music, theatre, gardening, gallery hopping and bookstore browsing, and the company of family and friends.

Ann Elizabeth Carson is a member of the Canadian Author's Association, the League of Canadian Poets, the Ontario Poetry Society, the Toronto Heliconian Club for professional women in the arts, and the Tower Poetry Society.

Illustrator Bio
Jennifer Kenneally

A graduate of several Fine Arts programs, lastly being Queen's University (Kingston), Jennifer has an Honours degree in Visual Arts and a B.Ed. with a focus on Arts Education. She has worked variously as a Registered Nurse, an actor and a teacher. Currently she owns and runs a thriving art school and studio in the creative and eclectic 'Beaches' area of Toronto, where she lives with her two crazily artistic daughters and an amazing and supportive fiancé. Artistically her twin passions are drawing and printmaking. Long having been fascinated by the aging face, and the singular beauty a lifetime of living gives to one's appearance, it is her hope and her mission to bring more images of older adults into the public consciousness.

Acknowledgements

My heartfelt thanks to the community that has helped in the making of this book:

To the women and men who shared their life stories with me over the years and to the 12 who agreed to let me present them here.

To Jennifer Kenneally, whose drawings lend wonderfully expressive faces to each story.

To Max Layton, Gianna Patriarca, Ellen Ryan, Olive Senior, and Linda Stitt, who write and encourage telling stories that "go against the grain."

To Anne Champagne, Arthur Joyce, Donna Langevin, John Parry, and Michael Salter, my gratitude for clarifying and honing the text with their alert and sensitive editorial wisdom. And to Margaret Lam for creative, calm, and invaluable online support.

My thanks to Marilyn Luciano, Paula Kirsh, Carolynn Bett, John and Sophie Rammell, Virginia Rock, Shirley Douglas, Mary Shirley-Thompson, Mairy Beam, Martha Saunders, Margo Little, Renia Tyminski, Pia and Wim Bouman, Grethe Jensen, Katherine Hill, Holly and Allen Briesmaster, Erin Harris, Pam Mordecai, and Bonni Kogos and to my children Michael, Meg, and Hilary Salter for their encouragement and enthusiasm along the way.

To publishers Shane Joseph and Sarah Jacob, who took a chance that there *are* people who want to read about aging and old age.

CPSIA information can be obtained
at www.ICGtesting.com
Printed in the USA
LVHW110850280419
615832LV00001B/82/P